TIME
Your Brain: A User's Guide

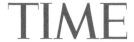

TIME

MANAGING EDITOR Richard Stengel
ART DIRECTOR Arthur Hochstein

Your Brain: A User's Guide

EDITOR Jeffrey Kluger
DESIGNER Sharon Okamoto
PICTURE EDITORS Hillary Raskin, Patricia Cadley
EDITORIAL PRODUCTION Lionel P. Vargas

TIME INC. HOME ENTERTAINMENT
PUBLISHER Richard Fraiman
GENERAL MANAGER Steven Sandonato
EXECUTIVE DIRECTOR, MARKETING SERVICES Carol Pittard
DIRECTOR, RETAIL & SPECIAL SALES Tom Mifsud
DIRECTOR, NEW PRODUCT DEVELOPMENT Peter Harper
ASSISTANT DIRECTOR, BOOKAZINE MARKETING Laura Adam
ASSISTANT PUBLISHING DIRECTOR, BRAND MARKETING Joy Butts
ASSOCIATE COUNSEL Helen Wan
BOOK PRODUCTION MANAGER Suzanne Janso
DESIGN & PREPRESS MANAGER Anne-Michelle Gallero
ASSOCIATE BRAND MANAGER Michela Wilde

SPECIAL THANKS TO:

Christine Austin, Natalia Brzostowska, Glenn Buonocore, Jim Childs, Susan Chodakiewicz, Jacqueline Fitzgerald, Rasanah Goss, Lauren Hall, Jennifer Jacobs, Brynn Joyce, Robert Marasco, Amy Migliaccio, Richard Prue, Brooke Reger, Ilene Schreider, Adriana Tierno, Alex Voznesenskiy, Sydney Weber, TIME Copy Desk, TIME Imaging

ISBN 10: 1-60320-094-0
ISBN 13: 978-1-60320-094-3
Library of Congress Control Number: 2009928291

We welcome your comments and suggestions about TIME Books. Please write to us at:
TIME Books, Attention: Book Editors, P.O. Box 11016, Des Moines, Iowa 50336-1016

If you would like to order any of our hardcover Collector's Edition books,
please call us at 1-800-327-6388
(Monday through Friday, 7 a.m.–8 p.m., or Saturday, 7 a.m.–6 p.m., C.T.).

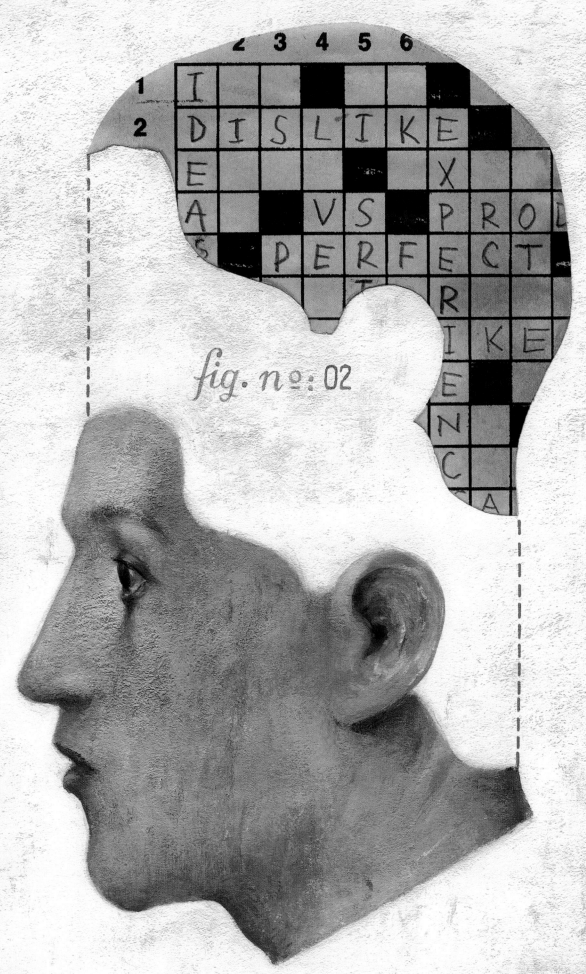

fig. nº: 02

Contents

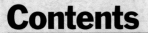

ILLUSTRATION BY DAVID PLUNKERT

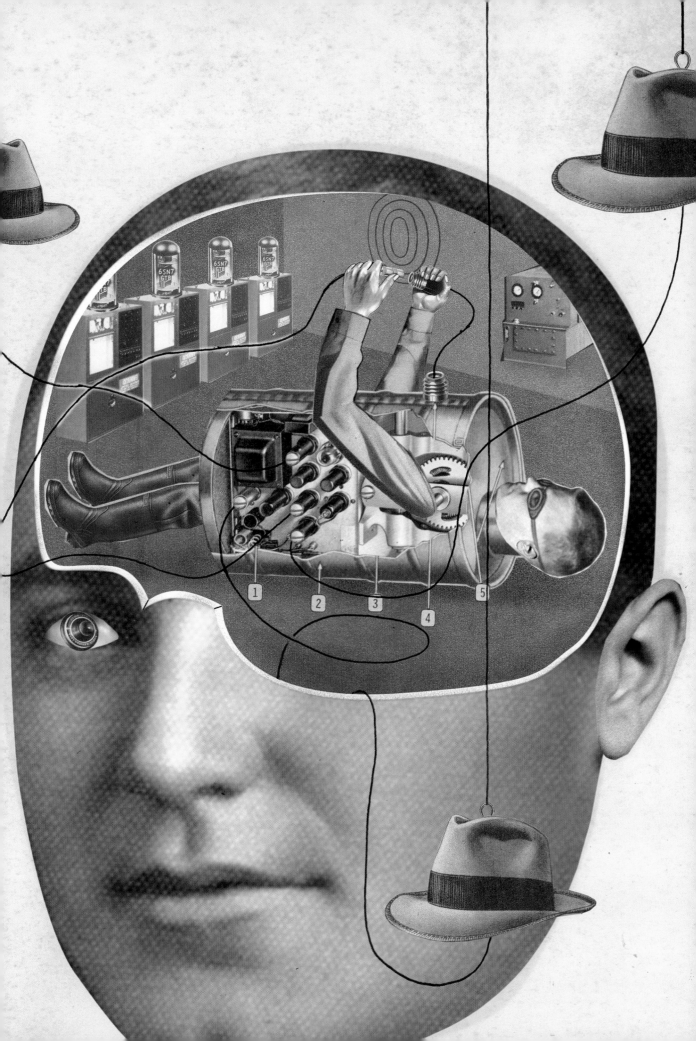

The Landscape Of the Mind

There's a universe inside your head—a place of pictures and passions, of songs and sorrows. It's everything you are—and it's an utter mystery

By Jeffrey Kluger

TRYING TO MAP THE BRAIN HAS ALWAYS BEEN CARTOGRAPHY FOR FOOLS. MOST of the other parts of the body reveal their workings with little more than a glance. The heart is self-evidently a pump; the lungs are clearly bellows. But the brain, which does more than any other organ, reveals least of all. The 3-lb. lump of wrinkled tissue—with no moving parts, no joints or valves—not only serves as the motherboard for all the body's other systems but also is the seat of your mind, your thoughts, your sense that you exist at all. You have a liver; you have your limbs. You are your brain.

The struggle of the mind to fathom the brain it inhabits is the most circular kind of search—the cognitive equivalent of M.C. Escher's famed lithograph of two hands drawing each other. But that has not stopped us from trying. In the 19th century, German physician Franz Joseph Gall claimed to have licked the problem with his system of phrenology, which divided the brain into dozens of "personality organs" to which the skull was said to conform. Learn to read those bony bumps and you could know the mind within. The artificial—and ultimately racist—field of craniometry made similar claims, relying on the overall size and shape of the skull to try to determine intelligence and moral capacity.

Modern scientists have done a far better job of things, dividing the brain into discrete regions with satisfyingly technical names—hypothalamus, caudate nucleus, neocortex—and mapping particular functions to particular sites. Here lives abstract thought; here lives creativity; here is emotion; here is speech. But what about here and here and here and here—all the countless places and ways the brain continues to baffle us? Here still be dragons.

Slowly, that is changing. As 21st century technology opens the brain to us like never before, accepted truths are becoming less true. The brain, we're finding, is indeed a bordered organ, subdivided into zones. But the lines are blurrier than we ever imagined. Lose your vision and the lobe that processed light may repurpose itself for sound. Suffer a stroke in the area that controls your right arm and another region may take over the job.

Specialized neurons are being found that allow us to mirror the behavior of people around us, helping us learn such primal skills as walking and eating as well as becoming social beings. The mystery of memory is being teased apart, exposing the way we store experiences.

Finally, and most elusively, we are learning something about consciousness itself—the ghost in the neural machine that gives you the sense of being in the moment, peering out at the world from the control room behind your eyes. If we can identify that cognitive kernel, can we one day endow a machine with it? But by isolating such a thing, do we in some way annihilate it too?

Human beings have always been brash enough to ask such questions but lacked the gifts to answer them. At last, we are acquiring that ability. What we can't yet know is whether we will use the remarkable things we're learning wisely or wantonly. ∎

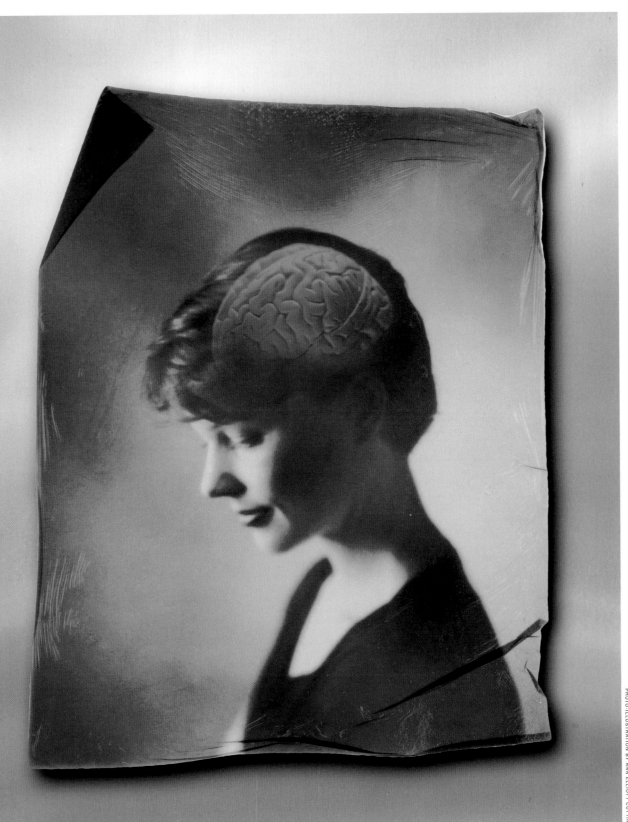

Five Paths To the Mind

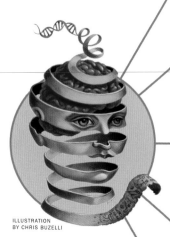

ILLUSTRATION
BY CHRIS BUZELLI

From gruesome
ancient rituals
to modern
pharmacology,
mankind has been
trying to discover
what's really going on
inside our heads.
A short history

BY JACKSON DYKMAN,
DAVID BJERKLIE AND ALICE PARK

Ancient beliefs What is the brain?

GRANGER
COLLECTION

5000 B.C.
Early evidence of
trephination, a
primitive brain surgery
in which a hole is cut
through the skull.
The practice, which
would persist through the
Middle Ages, was sometimes used to
treat seizures and headaches

2500 B.C.
Ancient Egyptians
believe the heart
is the source of
good and evil. They
consider the brain
an unimportant
organ and discard it
when mummifying
corpses

Anatomy How is the brain built?

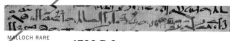

MALLOCH RARE
BOOK ROOM—
NEW YORK
ACADEMY OF
MEDICINE
LIBRARY

1700 B.C.
The 15-ft.-long Edwin Smith Surgical
Papyrus, a copy of Egyptian records
from 3000 B.C., includes the
earliest account of the anatomy of
the brain and describes 27 cases of
brain injury

300 B.C.
Alexandrian biologists
Herophilus, the "father
of anatomy," and
Erasistratus, his student,
are the first to rely on
dissection of the human
body to study the brain
and describe the nervous
system

Psychology How does the mind work?

1649
René Descartes
tackles the
philosophical
distinction
between mind
and body by proposing that
the immaterial soul enters
the body through the brain's
pineal gland

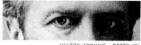

1890
William James publishes
Principles of Psychology, a
work widely hailed for its rich
and insightful descriptions of
human nature and behavior

HULTON ARCHIVE—GETTY (2)

Disorders Can we fix the brain?

1402
St. Mary of
Bethlehem is
England's first
hospital for the
mentally ill, and a
variant of its name,
bedlam, comes to
signify all psychiatric
facilities

1658
Johann
Jakof
Wepfer
proposes
that stroke is
caused by a
broken blood
vessel in the
brain

1883
Emil
Kraepelin
describes
schizo-
phrenia
and manic
depression

CULVER
PICTURES

Neuroscience What powers the brain?

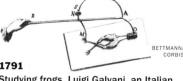

BETTMANN/
CORBIS

1791
Studying frogs, Luigi Galvani, an Italian
physiologist, is the first to propose that
some form of "animal electricity" secreted
by the brain drives nerve activity

1870
Camillo Golgi
develops a
staining method
that reveals
the detailed
structure of
sensory nerve
cells that feed
into the brain

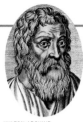

460-370 B.C.
Hippocrates describes epilepsy as a disorder of the brain, not a curse from the gods. He also believes the brain is the seat of intelligence and emotion

HULTON ARCHIVE
—GETTY

387-335 B.C.
Plato believes the brain controls intelligence and is "the divinest part of us." Aristotle, his student, believes the brain merely cools hot blood from the heart

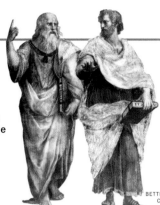

170 B.C.
Galen, physician to Roman gladiators, dissects the brains of sheep, monkeys, dogs and swine. He concludes that the cerebellum controls the muscles while the cerebrum processes the senses

BETTMANN/
CORBIS

1100-1500
Quacks practiced in sleight of hand go across Europe, claiming they can cure mental illnesses by removing "stones of madness" from the brain

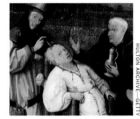

HULTON ARCHIVE—GETTY

1664
Thomas Willis, an Oxford professor, writes *Cerebri Anatome,* the most detailed description yet of the nervous system. Willis believes separate parts of the brain are responsible for thought and movement

1848
Railroad worker Phineas Gage's skull is pierced by an iron rod. He lives, but his personality reportedly changes, raising questions about how the brain's frontal regions affect behavior

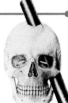

NATIONAL
LIBRARY OF
MEDICINE

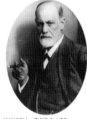

1899
Sigmund Freud argues in *Interpretation of Dreams* that dreams are windows to an otherwise inaccessible mind, "the royal road to the unconscious." It takes eight years to sell 600 copies

MANSELL—TIME & LIFE
PICTURES/GETTY

1903
In a famous experiment with dogs and dinner bells, Ivan Pavlov explores conditioned responses, an animal's involuntary reaction to stimuli, such as drooling at the sound of a bell

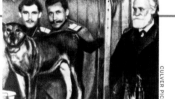

CULVER PICTURES

1938
B.F. Skinner describes how an animal's behavior can be engineered through positive and negative reinforcement

1906
Alois Alzheimer details presenile degeneration, which in 1910 becomes known as Alzheimer's disease

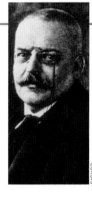

CORBIS

1936
Egas Moniz publishes a description of human frontal lobotomy as a treatment for psychosis

1949
Australian John Cade publishes findings that lithium is an effective treatment for bipolar disorder

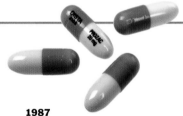

1987
Prozac is approved by the Food and Drug Administration as a treatment for depression

1936
Henry Hallett Dale, right, and Otto Loewi share the Nobel Prize for describing acetylcholine, a major chemical transmitter of nerve impulses

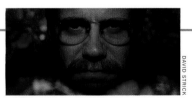

AP

1973
Michael Phelps, Edward Hoffman and Michael Ter Pogossian develop the positron-emission tomography scanner, which uses radioactive agents to image the brain

DAVID STRICK

1998
Fred Gage at the Salk Institute publishes a groundbreaking paper describing for the first time the ability of adult brain neurons to regenerate

2001
First gene-therapy trial to treat Alzheimer's disease

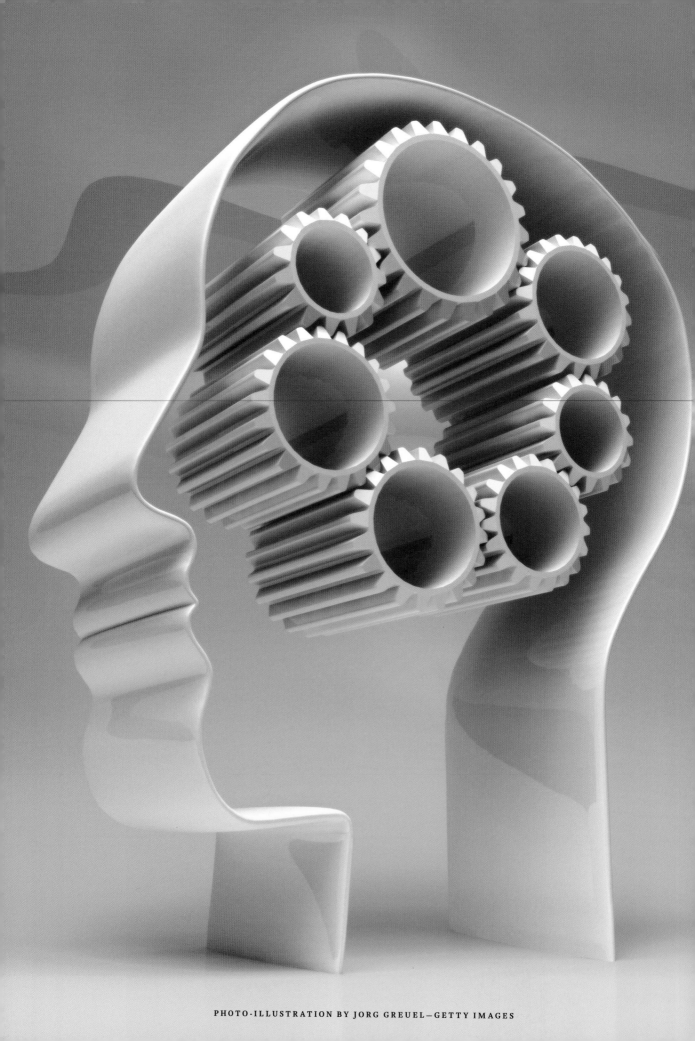

consci◉usness

Even the best computer in
the world has no idea that it
exists. You do. No one knows
what creates that ineffable
awareness that we're here, but
there are plenty of theories

The Riddle Of Knowing You're Here

You know what it feels like to be conscious—to observe the world from the control room behind your eyes. Now just try explaining how that works

BY STEVEN PINKER

THE YOUNG WOMAN HAD SURvived the car crash, after a fashion. In the five months since parts of her brain had been crushed, she could open her eyes but didn't respond to sights, sounds or jabs. In the jargon of neurology, she was judged to be in a persistent vegetative state. In crueler everyday language, she was a vegetable.

So picture the astonishment of British and Belgian scientists as they scanned her brain using a kind of MRI that detects blood flow to active regions. When they recited sentences, the parts involved in language lit up. When they asked her to imagine visiting the rooms of her house, the parts involved in navigating space and recognizing places ramped up. And when they asked her to imagine playing tennis, the regions that trigger motion joined in. Indeed, her scans were barely different from those of healthy volunteers.

Try to comprehend what it is like to be that woman. Do you appreciate the words and caresses of your distraught family while racked with frustration at your inability to reassure them that they are getting through? Or do you drift in a haze, springing to life with a concrete thought when a voice prods you, only to slip back into blankness? If we could experience this existence, would we prefer it to death? And if these questions have answers, would they change our policies toward unresponsive patients?

The report of this unusual case in 2006 was one more shock from a bracing new field, the science of consciousness. Questions once confined to theological speculations and late-night dorm-room bull sessions are now at the forefront of cognitive neuroscience. With some of the mysteries involved, a modicum of consensus is taking shape. With others, the puzzlement is so deep that answers may never be achieved. Some of our deepest convictions about what it means to be human could be shaken entirely.

It shouldn't be surprising that research on consciousness is alternately exhilarating and disturbing. No other topic is like it. As René Descartes noted, our own consciousness is the most indubitable thing there is. The major religions locate it in a soul that survives the body's death to receive its just reward or punishment or to meld into a global mind. For each of us, consciousness is life itself, the reason Woody Allen said, "I don't want to achieve immortality through my work. I want to achieve it by not dying." And the conviction that other people can suffer and flourish as each of us does is the essence of empathy and the foundation of morality.

To make scientific headway in a topic as tangled as

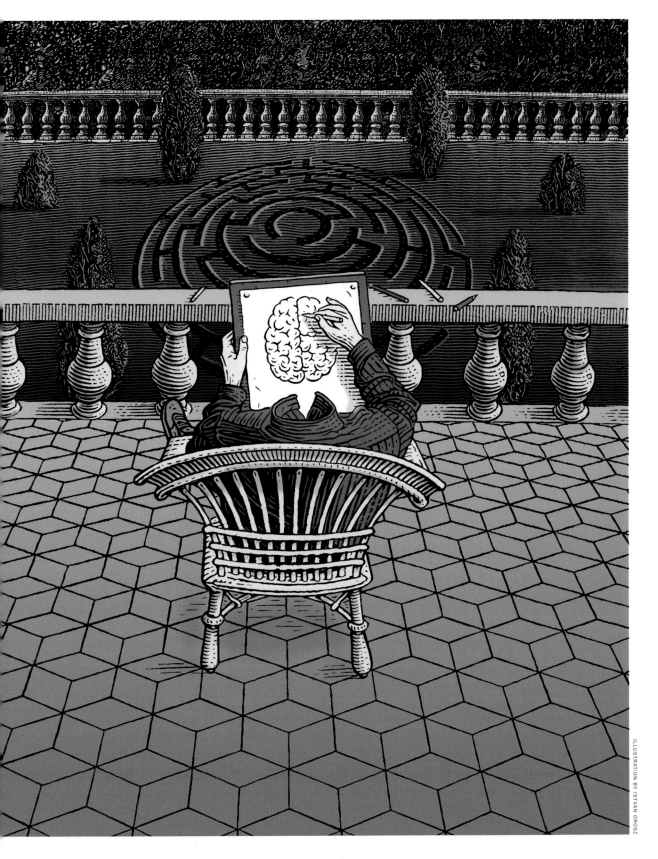

13

How to Read a Mind

This famous set of brain scans illustrates two things: **1)** a scanner can spot the difference between a brain recognizing a face and a brain recognizing a place and **2)** imagining faces or places lights up the same brain regions as actually seeing them. If your brain can't tell the difference between a real experience and an imagined one, how can you be sure you can?

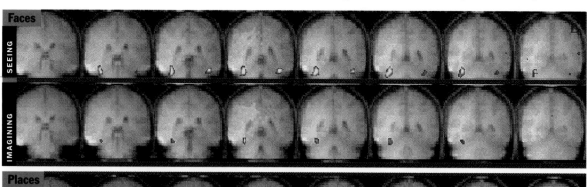

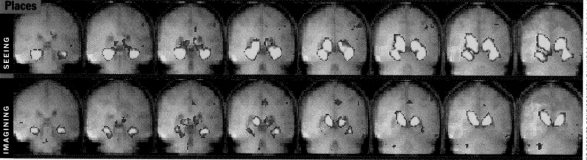

consciousness, it helps to clear away some misconceptions. Consciousness surely does not depend on language. Babies, many animals and patients robbed of speech are not insensate robots; they have reactions like ours that indicate that someone's home. Nor can consciousness be equated with self-awareness. At times we have all lost ourselves in music, exercise or sensual pleasure, but that is different from being knocked out cold.

What remains is not one problem about consciousness but two, which the philosopher David Chalmers has dubbed the Easy Problem and the Hard Problem. Calling the first one easy is an in-joke: it is easy in the sense that curing cancer or sending someone to Mars is easy. That is, scientists more or less know what to look for, and with enough brainpower and funding, they would probably crack the problem in this century.

What exactly is the Easy Problem? It's the one that

Freud made famous, the difference between conscious and unconscious thoughts. Some kinds of information in the brain—such as the surfaces in front of you, your plans for the day, your pleasures and peeves—are conscious. You can ponder them, discuss them and let them guide your behavior. Other kinds—like the control of your heart rate, the rules that order the words as you speak and the sequence of muscle contractions that allows you to hold a pencil—are unconscious. They must be in the brain somewhere because you couldn't walk and talk and see without them, but they are sealed off from your planning and reasoning circuits. The Easy Problem, then, is to distinguish conscious from unconscious mental computation, identify the proper correlates in the brain and explain why they evolved.

The Hard Problem, on the other hand, is why it *feels like* something to have a conscious process going on in

O'CRAVEN, K.M., AND KANWISHER, N. (2000). "MENTAL IMAGERY OF FACES AND PLACES ACTIVATES CORRE-SPONDING STIMULUS-SPECIFIC BRAIN REGIONS." JOURNAL OF COGNITIVE NEUROSCIENCE 12:1013.23

one's head—why there is first-person, subjective experience. Not only does a green thing appear different from a red thing, remind us of other green things and inspire us to say, "That's green" (the Easy Problem), but it also actually looks green: it produces an experience of sheer greenness that isn't reducible to anything else. As Louis Armstrong said in response to a request to define jazz, "When you got to ask what it is, you never get to know."

The Hard Problem is explaining how subjective experience arises from neural computation. The problem is hard because no one knows what a solution might look like or even whether it is a genuine scientific problem in the first place. And not surprisingly, everyone agrees that the Hard Problem (if it is a problem) remains largely a mystery.

Although neither the Hard nor the Easy Problem has been solved, neuroscientists agree on many features of both of them, and the feature they find least controversial is the one that many people outside the field find the most shocking. Francis Crick called it "the astonishing hypothesis"—the idea that our thoughts, sensations, joys and aches consist entirely of physiological activity in the tissues of the brain. Consciousness does not reside in an ethereal soul that uses the brain like a PDA; consciousness is the activity of the brain.

The brain, like it or not, is a machine. Scientists have come to that conclusion not because they are mechanistic killjoys but because they have amassed evidence that every aspect of consciousness can be tied to the brain. Using functional MRI, they can almost read people's thoughts from the blood flow in their brains. They can tell, for instance, whether a person is thinking about a face or a place or whether a picture the person is looking at is of a bottle or a shoe.

And consciousness can be pushed around by physical manipulations. Electrical stimulation of the brain during surgery can cause a person to have hallucinations that are indistinguishable from reality, such as a song playing in the room or a childhood birthday party. Chemicals that affect the brain, from caffeine and alcohol to Prozac and LSD, can profoundly alter how people think, feel and see. Surgery that severs the corpus callosum, separating the brain's two hemispheres (a treatment for epilepsy), spawns two consciousnesses within the same skull, as if the soul could be cleaved in two with a knife.

And when the physiological activity of the brain ceases, as far as anyone can tell, the person's consciousness goes out of existence. Attempts to contact the souls of the dead (a pursuit of serious scientists a century ago) turned up only cheap magic tricks, and near death experiences are merely symptoms of oxygen starvation in the brain and eyes.

Another startling conclusion from the science of consciousness is that the intuitive feeling we have that there's an executive "I" that sits in a control room of our brain, scanning the screens of the senses and pushing the buttons of the muscles, is an illusion. Consciousness turns out to consist of a maelstrom of events distributed across the brain. These events compete for attention, and as one process outshouts the others, the brain rationalizes the outcome after the fact and concocts the impression that a single self was in charge all along.

This illusion of voluntary actions is in part a result of noticing a correlation between what we decide and how our bodies move. The psychologist Dan Wegner studied the party game in which a subject is seated in front of a mirror while someone behind him extends his arms under the subject's armpits and moves his arms around, making it look as if the subject is moving his own arms. If the subject hears a tape telling the person behind him how to move (wave, touch the subject's nose and so on), he feels as if he is actually in command of the arms.

Why does consciousness exist at all, at least in the Easy Problem sense in which some kinds of information are accessible and others hidden? One reason is information overload. Just as a person can be overwhelmed today by the gusher of data coming in from electronic media, decision circuits inside the brain would be swamped if every curlicue and muscle twitch that was registered somewhere in the brain were constantly being reported to our conscious side. Instead, our working memory and spotlight of attention receive executive summaries of the events and states that are most relevant to updating an understanding of the world.

Another reason information may be sealed off from consciousness is tactical. Evolutionary biologist Robert Trivers has noted that people have a motive to sell themselves as beneficent, rational, competent agents. The best propagandist is the one who believes his own lies, ensuring that he can't leak his deceit through nervous

100 BILLION
The number of neurons in a human brain. Additional supporting material brings the total cell count closer to 1 trillion

125 MILLION
The number of visual receptors in each eye. Optical illusions show that the eyes compete for the brain's attention

6,000
The number of human genes, out of a total of 30,000, that are expressed in the brain and nowhere else— meaning our genome is 20% brain

twitches or self-contradictions. So the brain might have been shaped to keep compromising data away from the conscious processes that govern our interactions with other people. At the same time, it keeps the data around in unconscious processes to prevent the person from getting too far out of touch with reality.

What about the brain itself? You might wonder how scientists could even begin to find the seat of awareness in the cacophony of a hundred billion jabbering neurons. The trick is to see what parts of the brain change when a person's consciousness flips from one experience to another. In one technique, called binocular rivalry, vertical stripes are presented to the left eye, horizontal stripes to the right. The eyes compete for consciousness, and the person sees vertical stripes for a few seconds, then horizontal stripes, and so on.

A low-tech way to experience the effect yourself is to look through a paper tube at a white wall with your right eye and hold your left hand in front of your left eye. After a few seconds, a white hole in your hand should appear, then disappear, then reappear.

Monkeys experience binocular rivalry. They can learn to press a button every time their perception flips. Neuroscientist Nikos Logothetis found that the earliest way stations for visual input in the back of the brain barely budged as the monkeys' consciousness flipped from one state to another. Instead, it was a region that sits farther down the information stream that tracked the monkeys' awareness. What this means, according to a theory by Crick and his collaborator Christof Koch, is that consciousness resides only in the "higher" parts of the brain that are connected to circuits for emotion and decision-making.

Consciousness in the brain can be tracked not just in space but in time as well. Neuroscientists have long known that consciousness depends on certain frequencies of oscillation in an electroencephalograph (EEG). These brain waves consist of loops of activation between the cortex (the wrinkled surface of the brain) and the thalamus (the cluster of hubs at the center that serve as input-output relay stations). Large, slow, regular waves signal a coma, anesthesia or a dreamless sleep; smaller, faster, spikier ones correspond to being awake and alert. These waves may bind the activity in far-flung regions (one for color, another for shape, a third for motion, say) into a coherent conscious experience, a bit like radio transmitters and receivers tuned to the same frequency.

So neuroscientists are well on the way to identifying the neural correlates of consciousness, a part of the Easy Problem. But what about explaining how these events actually cause consciousness in the sense of inner experience—the Hard Problem?

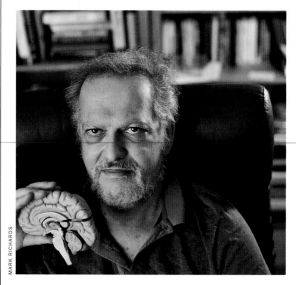

MARK RICHARDS

BERNARD BAARS

The Last Taboo

The topic of consciousness is much like sex was in the Victorian age. Scientifically, sex is just another part of biology, but in many societies, studying it violates a stern taboo. Once we begin to observe sexuality—or consciousness—a lot of the clouds of mystery seem to drift away.

That isn't to say that consciousness doesn't come with a great many stubborn mysteries. The topic of gravity, after all, is still mysterious four centuries after Isaac Newton first described it. But the difference is, there is no taboo about trying to understand gravity.

Baars is a senior fellow at the Neuroscience Institute. His most recent book is In the Theater of Consciousness

77%

The percentage of your brain that is cerebral cortex, where higher functions reside. In a rat's brain, it's 31%

On the Other Hand ...

Even the best explanation for consciousness is not the only one. Plenty of other scholars have tried to crack the riddle—and reached plenty of other conclusions

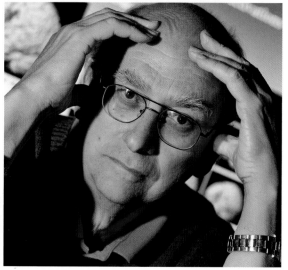

MICHAEL GAZZANIGA

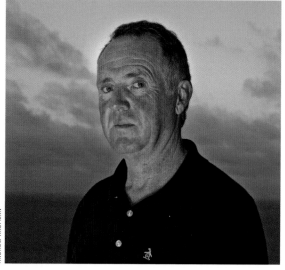

COLIN MCGINN

A Pipe Organ

Consciousness is an emergent property and not a process in and of itself. Our cognitive capacities, memories and dreams reflect distributed processes throughout the brain. The thousand conscious moments we have in a given day reflect one of our networks being up for duty. When it finishes, the next one pops up, and the pipe-organ-like device plays its tune all day long.

What makes emergent human consciousness so vibrant is that the human pipe organ has lots of tunes to play, whereas the rat's has few. And the more we know, the richer the concert.

Gazzaniga directs the SAGE Center for the Study of Mind at the University of California at Santa Barbara

The Unbridgeable Gulf

There appears to be what Wittgenstein called an "unbridgeable gulf" between the brain and the conscious mind. The paradox of the mind-body problem is that the cause of consciousness in the brain is not discoverable by inspecting the brain.

Nevertheless, consciousness is surely a natural biological product, as devoid of the otherworldly as digestion. So why is it so hard to fathom? The answer lies in ourselves: our brains have not evolved the equipment to resolve this mystery. They go blank when they try to understand how they produce the awareness that is our prized essence.

McGinn is a professor of philosophy at the University of Miami. His most recent book is Shakespeare's Philosophy

2.8

Weight, in pounds, of the average adult brain—or about 2% of body weight. A newborn's brain is a prodigious 8%

78%

The percentage of your brain that is water. Fats make up 12%, and proteins are 8%. The rest is salt and carbohydrates

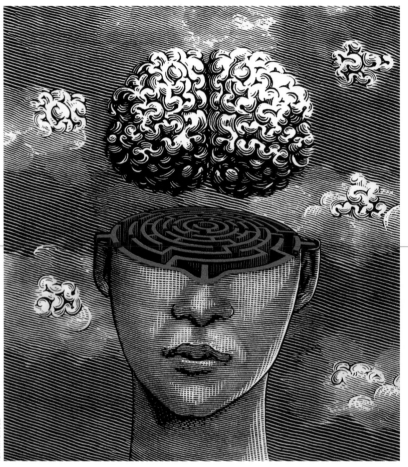

ISTVAN OROSZ

As philosophy students learn, nothing can force me to believe that anyone but me is conscious. The power to deny that other people have feelings is an all-too-common human vice

like finding out what wavelengths make people see green or how similar they say it is to blue, or what emotions they associate with it—boils down to information-processing in the brain and thus gets sucked back into the Easy Problem, leaving nothing else to explain. Most people react to this argument with incredulity because it seems to deny the ultimate undeniable fact: our own very real experiences.

The most popular attitude to the Hard Problem among neuroscientists is that it remains unsolved for now but will eventually succumb to research that chips away at the Easy Problem. Others are skeptical about this cheery optimism because none of the inroads into the Easy Problem brings a solution to the Hard Problem even a bit closer. Identifying awareness with brain physiology, they say, is a kind of "meat chauvinism" that would dogmatically deny consciousness to Lieut. Commander Data just because he doesn't have the soft tissue of a human brain. Identifying it with information-processing would go too far in the other direction and grant a simple consciousness to thermostats and calculators. Some mavericks, like the mathematician Roger Penrose, suggest the answer might someday be found in quantum mechanics. But to my ear, this amounts to the feeling that quantum mechanics sure is weird and consciousness sure is weird, so maybe quantum mechanics can explain consciousness.

And then there is the theory put forward by philoso-

To appreciate the hardness of the problem, consider how you could ever know whether you see colors the same way that I do. Sure, you and I both call grass green, but perhaps you see grass as having the color that I would describe, if I were in your shoes, as purple. Or ponder whether there could be a true zombie—a being who acts just like you or me but in whom there is no self actually feeling anything. This was the crux of a *Star Trek* plot in which officials wanted to reverse-engineer Lieut. Commander Data, and a furious debate erupted as to whether this was merely dismantling a machine or snuffing out a sentient life.

No one knows what to do with the Hard Problem. Some people may see it as an opening to sneak the soul back in, but this just relabels the mystery of "consciousness" as the mystery of "the soul"—a word game that provides no insight.

Many philosophers, like Daniel Dennett, deny that the Hard Problem exists at all. Speculating about zombies and inverted colors is a waste of time, they say, because nothing could ever settle the issue one way or another. Anything you could do to understand consciousness—

pher Colin McGinn that our vertigo when pondering the Hard Problem is itself a quirk of our brains. The brain is a product of evolution, and just as animal brains have their limitations, we have ours. Our brains can't hold a hundred numbers in memory, can't visualize seven-dimensional space and perhaps can't intuitively grasp why neural information processing observed from the outside should give rise to subjective experience on the inside. This is where I place my bet, though I admit that the theory could be demolished when an unborn genius—a Darwin or Einstein of consciousness—comes up with a flabbergasting new idea that suddenly makes it all clear to us.

Whatever the solutions to the Easy and Hard problems turn out to be, few scientists doubt that they will locate consciousness in the activity of the brain. For many nonscientists, this is a terrifying prospect. Not only does it strangle the hope that we might survive the death of our bodies, but it also seems to undermine the notion that we are free agents responsible for our choices. In his millennial essay "Sorry, but Your Soul Just Died," Tom Wolfe worried that when science has killed the soul, "the lurid carnival that will ensue may make the phrase 'the total eclipse of all values' seem tame."

My own view is that this is backward: the biology of consciousness offers a sounder basis for morality than the unprovable dogma of an immortal soul. It's not just that an understanding of the physiology of consciousness will reduce human suffering through new treatments for pain and depression. That understanding can also force us to recognize the interests of other beings—the core of morality.

As every student in Philosophy 101 learns, nothing can force me to believe that anyone except me is conscious. This power to deny that other people have feelings is not just an academic exercise but an all-too-common vice, as we see in the long history of human cruelty. Yet once we realize that our own consciousness is a product of our brains and that other people have brains like ours, a denial of other people's sentience becomes ludicrous. "Hath not a Jew eyes?" asked Shylock. Today the question is more pointed: Hath not a Jew—or an Arab, or an African, or a baby, or a dog—a cerebral cortex and a thalamus?

If that sounds mechanistic, if it makes us seem like transitory things, what of it? Think about why we sometimes remind ourselves that "life is short." It is an impetus to extend a gesture of affection to a loved one, to bury the hatchet in a pointless dispute, to use time productively rather than squander it. I would argue that nothing gives life more purpose than the realization that every moment of consciousness is a precious and fragile gift. ∎

ARE WE NOTHING BUT CLEVER ROBOTS?

Suppose Steven Pinker contracts a terrible progressive brain disease that destroys his nervous system from the outside in. But then neuroscience comes to the rescue, replacing each part of his nervous system as it disintegrates with an interfaced prosthesis made of silicone and wire.

Thanks to their success with the Easy Problems of consciousness, the scientists provide artificial substitutes for all Steve's brain powers. Moreover, he expresses satisfaction with his restored abilities and continues writing and speaking with humor and eloquence, delighting his friends and frustrating critics.

But can we really be sure he is expressing his satisfaction? His body may be just "expressing" his satisfaction. Although it appears that Steve believes he's alive and well, there is a possibility that his apparently animate body only "believes" it is alive.

The trouble with this hypothesis is that it declares its untestability at the outset. There is nothing Steve could do or say under any circumstances that would provide the slightest grounds for either dismissing or confirming the reality of his experience. There could not be an objective test to distinguish a clever robot from a conscious person. Now you have a choice: you can either cling to the Hard Problem, or you can shake your head in wonder and dismiss it. We've learned to do this before: it still seems that the sun goes around the earth, but we know better. It's not all that difficult, now that we've made so much progress on the Easy Problems. Just let go.

Daniel Dennett's most recent book is Breaking the Spell: Religion as a Natural Phenomenon

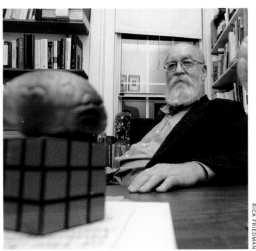

Why We Sleep

We do it every day—sometimes for 10 or more hours at a stretch—but that doesn't mean we know why. What good is sleep— and why do we need so much of it?

By Christine Gorman

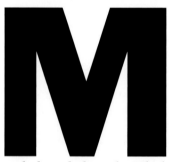

MAYBE YOU HAVE A BIG report due first thing in the morning. Or you're trying to deliver a truckload of fish before the wholesale market opens 150 miles away. Whatever the reason, you decide to stifle that yawn and push through the night. Whether or not you realize it, however, your brain has already started to check out.

After about 18 hours without sleep, your reaction time begins to slow. You start to experience bouts of microsleep—moments when you zone out for anywhere from two to 20 seconds and drift out of your lane or find that you have to keep rereading the same passage. Your reaction time, studies show, will eventually be about the same as that of someone who is legally drunk.

Although you may get a second wind with the rising of the sun, the longer you stay up, the more your condition deteriorates. "By the second night, oh, my goodness, it's extremely dramatic," says David Dinges, a sleep expert at the University of Pennsylvania School of Medicine. "You fall massively off the cliff."

All through the animal kingdom, sleep ranks right up there with food, water and sex for the survival of the spe-

cies. Yet scientists still don't know precisely what sleep is for. Is it to refresh the body? Not really. Researchers have yet to find any vital biological function that sleep restores. Is it to refresh the mind? That's closer to the mark. The brain benefits from a good night's sleep. But there has never been much agreement among sleep researchers about what form that benefit takes. That's slowly changing. Most of the new science of sleep has emerged quite recently, with new scanning equipment that allows scientists to take increasingly detailed pictures of the sleeping brain, down to the individual neuron. "In the past year or two, everything seemed to click together," says Dr. Giulio Tononi, a neurobiologist and psychiatrist at the University of Wisconsin at Madison.

Even before the recent insights, scientists knew that most mammals, with the possible exception of dolphins and whales, cycle between two phases of sleep. One is characterized by rapid eye movement—the famous REM sleep. The other is called simply non-REM sleep.

The EEGs of people in REM sleep show lots of brain activity—and if you wake them up during it, they will tell you that they have just been dreaming. Despite the mythology that surrounds dream imagery, the consensus among sleep researchers is that dreaming is nothing more than the random recycling of the day's events.

For years, sleep researchers focused most of their attention on REM sleep, but they kept running into blank

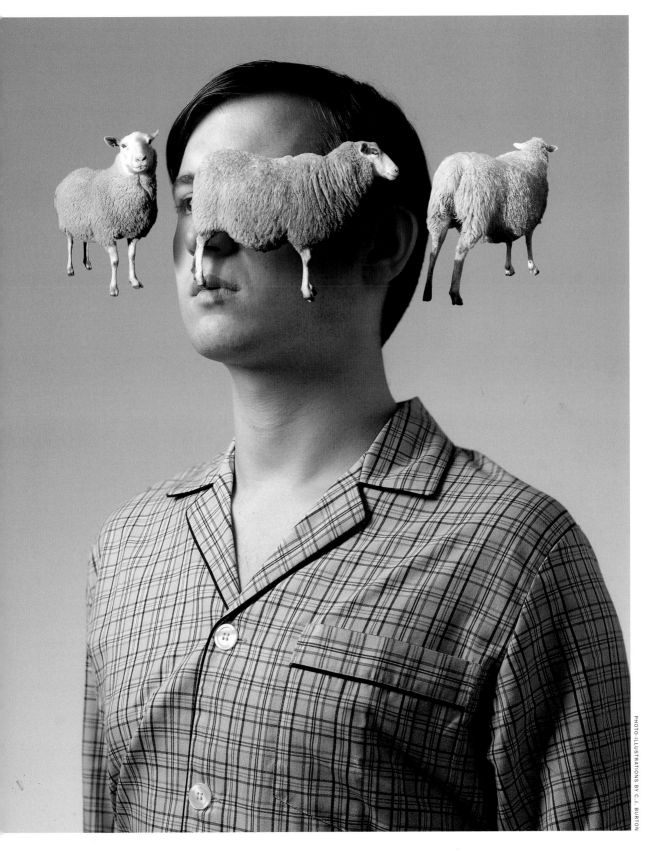

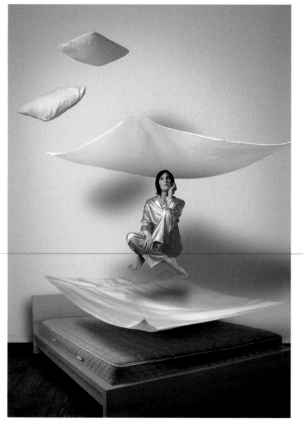

In one study, subjects who learned a task at night were 40% more accurate and 20% faster when they were tested after sleeping than those who learned the task in the morning and were tested later in the day

walls. Early work that tried to link REM sleep to learning foundered when scientists discovered that their test subjects could remember long lists of new words or facts whether or not they got any REM sleep. Things became clearer in 1994, when researchers at the Weizmann Institute of Science in Rehovot, Israel, suggested that your ability to recognize patterns on a computer screen is directly tied to the amount of REM sleep you get. Such skills depend on something called procedural memory, which is needed for any task that requires repetition and practice.

Over the past couple of years, Robert Stickgold, a cognitive neuroscientist at Harvard Medical School, has teamed up with Matthew Walker of Boston's Beth Israel Deaconess Medical Center to investigate sleep's effects on procedural memory for motor skills. They asked right-handed test subjects to type a sequence of numbers with their left hand as fast as they could. No matter what time of day they learned the task, their accuracy improved 60% to 70% after six minutes of practice. When subjects who learned the sequence in the morning were retested 12 hours later, they didn't significantly improve. But when those who learned the sequence in the evening were retested following a night's sleep, they were 15% to 20% faster and 30% to 40% more accurate.

New technology is leading to more insights. Research

by Bruce McNaughton, a psychologist and physiologist at the University of Arizona, in Tucson, has shown that many of the same neurons that fire during the daytime—say, when a rat is learning to navigate a maze—are reactivated during the REM stage of sleep. "Basically, the brain is reviewing its recently stored data," McNaughton says. Eventually the brain consolidates those patterns.

Perhaps, then, that's what sleep really is—repeated cycles that allow you to learn new tricks without forgetting old ones. Of course, none of that explains why you have to be unconscious for it to happen. Maybe it's just easier not to be awake while the work is going on. "It's like you're leaving your house, and the workmen come in to renovate," suggests Terry Sejnowski, a computational neurobiologist at the Salk Institute in La Jolla, Calif.

Perhaps it's simpler than that. Perhaps we sleep merely because our brains need the break. Like the rest of the body, the brain runs on glucose. Using computerized scanners that provide images in real time, Dr. Gregory Belenky of Washington State University at Spokane has shown that the brain's ability to use glucose drops off dramatically after being awake 24 hours. That's like being hungry and having a cupboard full of food but not being able to eat it. Sleep may correct the problem.

Whatever sleep turns out to be for, researchers admit they still don't know how much we need. There's a mythological power in the popular eight-hour target, but myth might be just what it is. Surveys suggest that we get less sleep than folks did a century ago, but that's not necessarily a problem. "Our sleeping environments are better than they ever have been," says Jim Horne, director of the Sleep Research Centre at Loughborough University in England. So how much sleep should you get? Most researchers are practical. "If you feel sleepy the following day," says Pierre-Hervé Luppi, Ph.D., of the University of Lyons in France, "it means you're not sleeping enough." You don't have to know what sleep is for to know that it's good for you. ∎

Perchance to Dream

Whether you spend the day at hard labor or just lazing about, you're going to get drowsy. That's your brain telling you it needs a rest. A tired body can recover by reducing activity, but a tired cerebral cortex must have sleep. Here's how your brain and body interact through the night

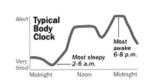

WIDE AWAKE

Your brain is constantly processing input from the senses; about one-third of that information arrives via the eyes. All this daily stimulation makes you feel tired, usually at regular intervals

Brain waves show constant, rapid activity

Alert **Typical Body Clock** *Most awake 6-8 p.m. Most sleepy 2-6 a.m. Very tired* — Midnight · Noon · Midnight

1. DROWSINESS

Usually lasts 10 to 30 minutes

You're dozing off, disengaging from the world. Your muscles relax, but sometimes you may experience *hypnic jerks*—sudden spasms that wake you up, often with the feeling of falling

Brain activity begins to slow

2. LIGHT SLEEP

About half of sleep time

Your body temperature drops, and your heart rate slows. Brain waves display sporadic *spindles* and *K complexes*, believed to be the mind maintaining sleep by blocking out exterior disturbances

Spindle   K complex

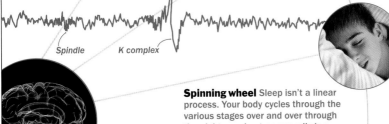

Spinning wheel Sleep isn't a linear process. Your body cycles through the various stages over and over through the night—and not necessarily in a particular order

3. DEEP SLEEP

Along with deepest sleep, makes up 25% of sleep time

This is the beginning of restful sleep, also known as *delta sleep* because it's denoted by slower brain waves. Physiologically, this stage is indistinguishable from deepest sleep

Frequent K complexes

4. DEEPEST SLEEP

This is the sleep your body needs the most when you've been awake too long. It's also the stage during which most brain recovery is thought to occur. Waking up from this type of sleep can be briefly disorienting

Continuous K complexes

5. REM SLEEP

Occurs about every 90 minutes throughout sleep cycle

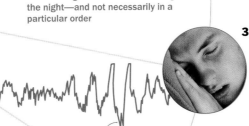

Named for its characteristic rapid eye movements, this is when vivid dreaming occurs. Blood pressure rises, and breathing becomes erratic. Your brain is very active, almost as if you're awake, but your body is paralyzed—your muscles (other than those that maintain heartbeat and respiration) completely shut down

Similar pattern to wakened state

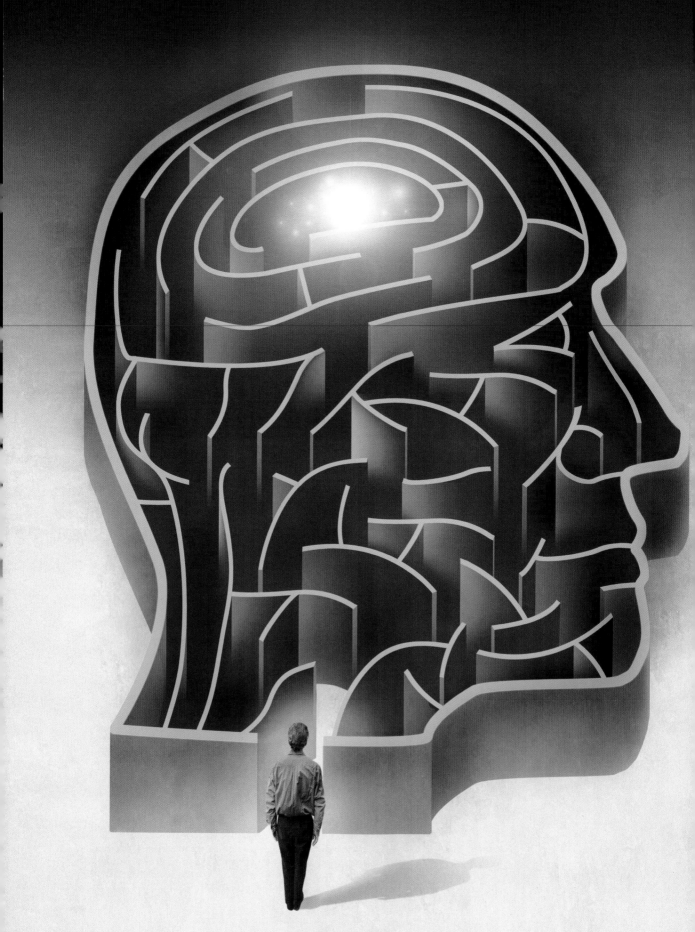

PHOTO-ILLUSTRATION BY MATT MAHURIN

learn+ing

You're born with nature's best computer inside your
head—and you spend a lifetime adding programs

Language And the Baby Brain

Learning to speak was the hardest thing you ever did, yet you had the job mastered by the time you were in kindergarten. How did you manage such a feat?

BY JEFFREY KLUGER

THERE IS NO REAL REASON YOU should be able to talk. You began learning almost as soon as you were born, and you pretty much had it nailed before you even started school. That, however, doesn't mean it makes any sense that you can do it at all.

Consider the numbers: We start life nonlingual. Within 18 months, we have a core working vocabulary of 50 words we can pronounce and 100 or so more we understand. By the time we're 3, we have about 1,000 words at our command and are constructing often elaborate sentences. By our sixth birthday, our vocabulary has exploded to 6,000 words—meaning that we've learned, on average, three new words every day since birth. Mastering good conversational English requires about 50,000 words, and that includes those that are formal and endorsed by the dictionary. There are thousands of other idioms and fixed expressions—*day by day, around the block, end of the week, top of the ninth, fending off, touch and go, bundle up, buckle down* and on and on. And what about children

who learn a second or third language, doubling or tripling the information they must collect and store and keep from commingling?

There are few better places to begin understanding the phenomenon of human speech than April Benasich's neuroscience lab at the Center for Molecular and Behavioral Neuroscience on the campus of Rutgers University in Newark, N.J. On any particular day, there are a lot of smart, busy people at work in Benasich's lab, but the nimblest brains in residence usually belong to the handful of people who are too young to have any real idea of why they're there.

Take Jack, who's just over a year old. While his mother holds him on her lap inside a small soundproof room, Benasich, a clinical psychologist and the director of the center, fits him with a soft, netted hat shot through with 64 electrodes. When the hookup is done, Benasich's assistants throw a switch, and a computer-generated voice begins to speak into the room. It doesn't say much—just three syllables, which it repeats in random order and at various intervals: *da, ta,* and then another, slightly different *ta,* flattened a bit, the way it is in well-accented Spanish. To the adult ear, the sounds are indistinguishable. But Jack does not have an adult's ear; he has a 13-month-old's ear, and that's a very different instrument. As he listens, the electrodes sense changes in what is known as the brain's evoked response potential (ERP),

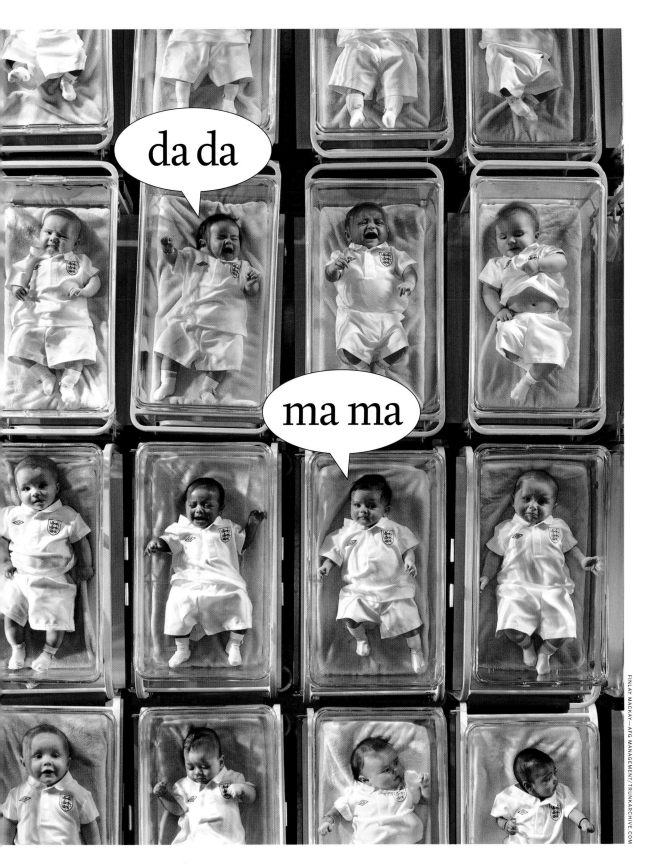

electrical hiccups indicating not only that the speech and hearing centers have heard the syllables, but also that the differences have been distinguished.

"It's a remarkable thing to watch," says Benasich. "Hearing the differences in pronunciation like that requires you to make distinctions in sounds that take only 35 milliseconds to play out—and often a lot less."

The roots of such prodigious talent lie in the design of the baby's brain. All human brains contain roughly the same number of individual neurons—about 100 million. But a baby's brain is wired differently, with any individual neuron connected to as many as 15,000 other neurons; each of those 15,000 then branches out in 15,000 other ways. Across the entire body of the brain, this adds up to well over 1 quadrillion cellular links. Adult brains have about a third fewer links per neuron, or only about 10,000.

It's this extra wiring that enables a baby's brain to learn languages so easily, and the key to that gift is, partly, processing speed. If incoming information bombards the brain too fast, all the data bits will eventually run together, in much the same way music played at high speed becomes atonal gibberish or a train whizzing by turns into a blur. The better you can distinguish each word, syllable and sound coming in, the better you'll learn to speak.

To clock how fast the ear processes word bits, Benasich has babies listen to tones and phonemes separated by a 300-millisecond gap—fast by most standards but slow to the flash drive of the brain. Benasich then steadily shortens the gap, all the while monitoring the babies with ERP readouts. Consistently, her studies show that the babies' brains have no trouble keeping up all the way down to 35 milliseconds, the point at which the length of the gap grows shorter than the length of the phoneme. Even then, the babies keep pace, getting down to an 8-millisecond spread before finally going deaf to the breaks.

"The babies eventually fall behind not because they lose interest or because the brain's wiring gets overloaded," says Benasich. "Rather, it's the individual neurons that become overwhelmed. Every time a neuron hears a tone, it fires. But before it can register a new tone, it has to get back to chemical baseline. Eventually, the neurons simply can't do it fast enough."

The younger a brain is, the faster it can go before the neurons give up this way. Parents raising multilingual children already know that the earlier they introduce a child to a second or third language, the less effort it takes to acquire. New studies are helping measure that phenomenon and are revealing that age differences of just a few months can make big differences in learning.

At the University of Washington at Seattle, psychologist Andrew Meltzoff and speech and hearing specialist Patricia Kuhl devised a revealing experiment in which a group of babies, all just a few months old, were brought in for half-hour play sessions three times a week for four weeks. All the children were from English-speaking homes, and all were supervised in the sessions by a caregiver who read to them and talked to them. In some cases, the caregivers spoke only English; in other cases, they spoke only Mandarin. At the end of the month, the babies were brought back in.

This time, there was no caregiver, and the babies were allowed to play on their own. As they did, a loudspeaker nearby emitted a series of random, computer-generated sounds such as *oo* and *ee*. Buried within the tones were occasional Mandarin phonemes. Babies who had been with the Mandarin-speaking caregivers looked toward the loudspeaker when they heard those familiar sounds, indicating that they'd retained what they'd learned in the play sessions. Babies with English-speaking caregivers heard nothing meaningful.

Brain-wave mapping like that done in Benasich's

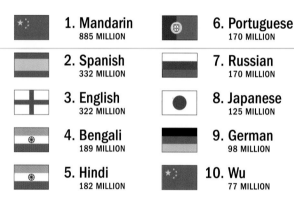

TOP 10 TONGUES
Mandarin has the most speakers—by a lot

1. Mandarin 885 MILLION	6. Portuguese 170 MILLION
2. Spanish 332 MILLION	7. Russian 170 MILLION
3. English 322 MILLION	8. Japanese 125 MILLION
4. Bengali 189 MILLION	9. German 98 MILLION
5. Hindi 182 MILLION	10. Wu 77 MILLION

6,000
Number of words in your vocabulary by the time you're 6 years old, meaning you've learned three new words per day since birth

50,000
Number of words required to speak advanced English. There are thousands more figures of speech, like *buckle down* and *raise the roof*

15,000
Number of connections each neuron in a baby's brain can make. In adults, it's 10,000, one reason babies are better at learning languages

Languages Around the World

Human beings currently speak 6,800 different tongues, with new ones dying and being born all the time. Papua New Guinea is the world's most polyglot place, with 820 languages

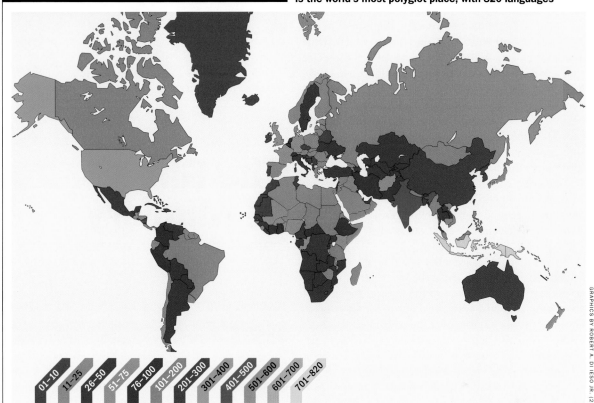

01–10 | 11–25 | 26–50 | 51–75 | 76–100 | 101–200 | 201–300 | 301–400 | 401–500 | 501–600 | 601–700 | 701–820

GRAPHICS BY ROBERT A. DI IESO JR. (2)

lab confirmed what the babies' behavior was showing. Significantly, however, not all the babies who heard the Mandarin heard it equally well. Generally, the older the babies were when they started the study, the better they did, but only until they reached 9 months or so. At that point, the door to language slowly began to swing shut. Babies exposed to Mandarin for the first time at 1 year routinely performed less well than kids half their age or younger. "Linguistically," Kuhl wrote in her book *The Scientist in the Crib,* "children start out as citizens of the world, but they don't stay that way."

Impressive as the results of Kuhl's study were, not all the trials were a success. For one thing, the babies pick up the sounds of the alien language only if the person speaking it to them is in the room. When the test was repeated, but this time the caregiver reading the stories and doing the cooing was merely a video, the babies tuned out completely. Yet a video teacher works just fine if the skill being taught is manual, not linguistic. Babies who watch a tape of an adult playing with an unfamiliar toy will later recognize that toy in a pile of other ones and begin to play with it properly. Since language is such a social skill, research-

ers believe, it takes real social interaction—including eye contact and pointing—for it to be learned properly.

If babies are such natural linguists, why don't we all retain that skill? Why shouldn't the neuronal power of the brain we had at birth—its "exuberant growth" of synapses, as Benasich calls it—stay with us for a lifetime?

One reason might be that this kind of streamlining is simply what complex systems do. Corporations, committees, cities, brains all start out with the most sprawling and varied structure they can in order to give themselves the most flexibility possible. You can't tell exactly what direction your work will take you in until you actually begin doing it, so you must be able to do it all. Over time, as the system becomes more adept, it begins a process of self-consumption—a sort of refinement by reduction—digesting and shedding parts of itself in order to move toward a state of greater efficiency.

In the case of language, this might be especially important. The only way to stabilize a child's main language (or for multilinguals, the main two or three) is to begin hardening the brain around familiar sounds and syntaxes, filtering out distracting ones that will not be needed.

Lotus Lin, a Taiwanese-born researcher in Kuhl's lab, has looked into that process, conducting studies in which Japanese and English-speaking American adults listen to recordings of *r* and *l* sounds while their brains are scanned with magnetic encephalography. In the American brains, sensitive to the two letters, a discrete neuronal cluster lights up, representing the precise spot at which the sound is heard and identified. In the Japanese brains, which learned a language that makes no real distinction between the two sounds, there is a much larger and more diffuse splatter of activity, with neuronal firing beginning in the same small region and spreading outward, as if the brain is groping for a way to identify what it is hearing.

"We conduct test runs first," says Lin, "exposing both sets of listeners to *ba* and *wa* sounds. Since these phonemes are used in both languages, all of the subjects hear them equally well. It's only when we try the *r* and *l* that you see the difference."

This cross-cultural atonality would be less meaningful if it were simply a quirk of the Asian ear. But Westerners are just as tone-deaf to the musical cadences of Cantonese. Russians are baffled at the wholly irreproducible way Italians pronounce the *gl* blend. Greeks can't make sense of the diphthongs of Thais. If you don't learn it early, the rule seems to be, you'll never learn it at all.

Another reason we scale down our language ability as we age may be the simple matter of energy conservation. Maintaining the operation of 1 quadrillion synapses burns a lot of calories. It's possible, some researchers believe, that the neural complexity we're born with is simply not energetically sustainable throughout our lives—particularly as we get older and the ravenous consumption of food that fueled our early physical growth slows.

"We were a nutritionally marginal species early on," says psychologist William Greenough, an expert on brain development at the University of Illinois at Urbana-Champaign, "and a synapse is a very costly thing to support. The consequences of getting language wrong are so high that it's vitally important to get it right, which means you need a big system at first. Then you can prune it back."

As we do, the language door closes and our polyglot gift vanishes almost completely. In the long arc of a lifetime, this is not all bad. The command of a preferred language that we improve and refine over decades of speaking is far more nuanced, far more lyrical than what any child could begin to approach. Hamlet and Huckleberry Finn, after all, did not spring from the pen of a toddler. Even if we mourn the linguistic abilities we lose as we age, this focused excellence is a triumph of its own. ∎

The Gift Of Mimicry

Brains brim with original ideas, but they also love to imitate. Neurons constantly watch what other people are doing and mime it themselves. That's how we learn

ONCE YOU'VE SEEN A TARANTULA CRAWL along the skin of James Bond's shoulder, you're not likely to forget it. Even if you've never squirmed through the iconic scene in the classic *Dr. No,* the mere description of it is likely to make your skin crawl just a little.

That oddly personal, oddly tactile reaction is not only the result of deft moviemaking; it's also the handiwork of your somatosensory cortex—the place in your brain where real tickles are processed. As Bond feels the tarantula, his somatosensory cortex crackles with nasty signals and, in a smaller way, yours does too. Such neurological empathy would not be possible without the help of specialized brain cells known as mirror neurons.

Mirror neurons are found all over the brain, and they're responsible for a whole range of phenomena. When a mother opens her mouth and a newborn imitates her, mirror neurons are at work. When someone finds forgotten leftovers in the refrigerator and recoils at the sight and smell of them and you recoil too, that's also mirror neurons. Mirror neurons are even involved when you look at a sculpture like Bernini's *Rape of Proserpina* in the Borghese Gallery in Rome. "Even though the statue is made of marble, one of the coldest materials on earth, it conveys a

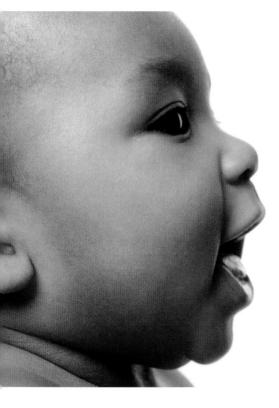
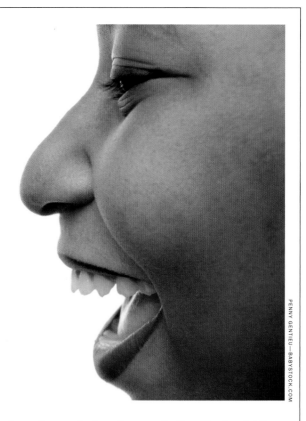

vivid impression of carnality," says neuroscientist Vittorio Gallese of the University of Parma.

Under a microscope, mirror neurons look like other neurons. What makes them special is the web of connections that links these neurons in the motor and sensory systems to the limbic centers that process visceral and emotional reactions. And while some of these connections may well be in place at birth, they are, neuroscientists think, vastly expanded through experience. A baby smiles. Her mother smiles back. Click. The brain sets up a circuit.

Gallese was part of a team that published some of the earliest work on mirror neurons back in the 1990s, when he and his colleagues were conducting brain studies on macaques and noticed something odd: the monkeys would be sitting still, doing nothing in particular, when a researcher would pick up raisins or sunflower seeds. At that point, the neurons the monkeys would use if they were engaging in the same task began buzzing. It was as if the macaques were mentally mirroring the action they observed.

All manner of experiments have yielded similar results. A study conducted in the Netherlands revealed that a discrete patch of the somatosensory cortex lit up both when human subjects felt their legs being brushed

by a glove and when they watched a video in which an actor's legs were brushed. A British study showed that the mere thought that a loved one's hand is receiving an electric shock lights up many of the same brain areas as shocks that are directly experienced. A U.S. study revealed that mirror neurons can even calibrate their responses up and down: volunteers watched a pair of videos, one showing a hand reaching for a brimming teacup next to a plate of cookies, another showing a hand reaching for an empty cup surrounded by crumbs. In both cases, mirror neurons fired in the parietal cortex, where motor control is processed, but in the first case they fired more powerfully, since the goal—fresh cookies, hot tea—was more appealing.

All this mimicry inside our heads is much more than a neural party trick. Researchers believe mirror neurons may be a key to the way human beings learn speech, signal meaning to one another and develop primal feelings of empathy. "When you watch a movie," says neuroscientist Christian Keysers of University Medical Center Groningen in the Netherlands, who, along with his colleagues, conducted the glove-brushing study, "you don't think to yourself, Now the hero is smiling, so he must be happy. Through the mirror system, you just know it." —*By J. Madeleine Nash*

The Most Important Sex Organ

Think men's and women's bodies are different? Try taking a peek inside our skulls. Our brains start out different in the womb—and grow only more so as we age

By Lori Oliwenstein

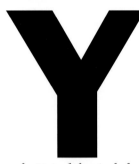

YOUR BRAIN HAS A GENDER. If you're a guy, you have a guy's brain; if you're a woman, you're a woman from top to bottom.

Sounds obvious, right? After all, every cell of a woman's body carries two X chromosomes; every cell of a man's body carries an X and a Y. And that includes brain cells. Plus, the sex hormones that constantly course through our bodies don't bypass our brains. Why wouldn't this unending hormonal bath work its transformative magic there too?

And yet, until fairly recently, brains were thought of as asexual and interchangeable—more like hearts or livers than like breasts and genitals. Very one-size-fits-all. Over the past decade, however, brain scientists have come to appreciate what scientists studying other aspects of gender have learned—that some of the most critical differences between men and women are hidden not beneath the zippers of our jeans but inside the twists of our genes.

"The evidence is overwhelming that sex influences brain and nervous-system function," says neurobiologist Larry Cahill of the University of California at Irvine, "and that it does so from the level of the whole human all the way down to the level of single neurons in petri dishes."

At the upper end of that scale is the undeniable fact that men's brains are, on average, 8% to 10% larger than women's brains—and that they're packed more densely with nerve cells. Women's brains, on the other hand, are roomier; there's more space between neurons, allowing for a greater number of connections to be made and thus more networking to be done.

Female brains also tend to mature sooner, a fact that anyone roaming the halls of a junior high school knows. A 2007 study led by the National Institutes of Health (NIH) looked at brain development in people ages 3 to 27 and found that girls' brains reach their maximum volume by the time girls are about 10½, while boys' brains lag a full four years behind, hitting their peak when boys are 14½.

If you narrow your focus—look at, say, the corpus callosum (the cable that connects the two hemispheres of the brain) or the temporal lobe (which governs such critical functions as semantics and perception)—those age ranges and the gap between them grow or shrink, but the girl-first sequence never changes. The most critical difference might be in the brain's gray matter—the tissue in which real thinking gets done—as opposed to the white matter, which is mostly nerves and fatty sheathing. The volume of gray matter peaks in girls one to two years earlier than in boys, corresponding nicely to the average age difference in the onset of puberty.

Individual brain structures differ not just in rates of

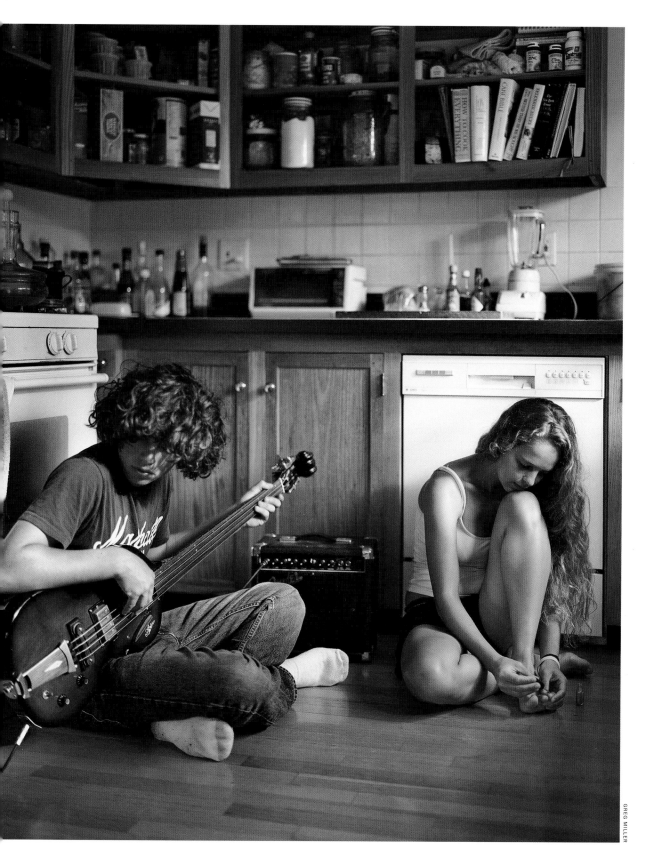

14½ The age at which boys' brains reach peak size. Boys excel at visualizing three-dimensional objects in space

development but in their overall size relative to the rest of the brain—and they do so in ways that provoke all manner of hot political debate. Two of the key language centers are larger in women than in men, for instance, which seems to confirm the general belief that girls are better linguists than boys. Similarly, a brain section linked to mental-arithmetic abilities is larger in men than in women, which—like it or not—offers some anatomical support for the idea that boys are better in math. In 1991 the prosaically named third interstitial nucleus of the anterior hypothalamus became the world's most famous neuron clump when neuroscientist Simon LeVay showed that it is half as big in women and homosexual men as it is in heterosexual men. And then there are these other in-your-cranium differences to consider:

■ Women are more likely than men to be clinically depressed, while autism is disproportionately a disorder of males.
■ Women process pain signals in the parts of their brains that handle emotion, while men shuttle these same messages to the more analytic regions.
■ Women excel at fine-motor tasks like putting pegs in small holes, while men are hard to beat at target-directed activities like darts and archery.
■ Despite the anatomical differences in math-linked brain regions, women are better at straightforward arithmetic (adding, subtracting and so forth); men are better at reasoning their way through a math problem.

Men also have the definite upper lobe when it comes to tasks like envisioning how a three-dimensional object will look when it's rotated in space. This mental party trick is actually "the single largest sex difference in cognition that's been discovered," notes psychologist David Moore, who directs the Claremont Infant Study Center at Pitzer College in California.

That makes it the perfect tool to use when trying to glimpse some of the earliest signs of sex differences. And, indeed, Moore's studies of mental-rotation abilities in infants have shown that when boys as young as 3 months are shown an object that they've seen before but that has been rotated to a new position, they'll give it only a cursory glance, indicating that they already know what it is. Girls

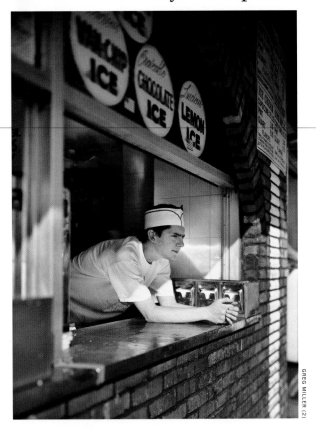

GREG MILLER (2)

will stare at the rotated object longer, indicating that it looks new to them. It's uncertain why this difference exists, but other studies have found that the parietal lobe, which is where this rotational ability lives in the brain, does have more surface area in men than in women.

All this notwithstanding, differences in brain structure and the traits they confer never fall neatly into silos—boys-have-this and girls-do-that categories that would explain everything as a simple matter of cerebral architecture. Just as gender doesn't define who you are, neither does it define what your brain is or what you as an individual are capable of learning or doing.

"People tend to think about sex differences in terms of black and white, Mars and Venus," Cahill notes. But while women indeed have higher rates of depression, for example—perhaps because of generally lower levels of the neurotransmitter serotonin—there are plenty of men

10½ The age at which girls' brains reach peak volume. Most girls excel at language earlier than boys

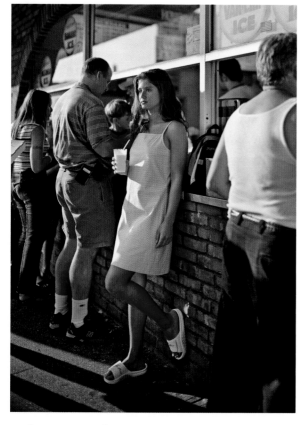

on therapists' couches. And although studies have shown that men's cognitive abilities decline more quickly with age than women's, there are plenty of sharp old guys out there—and plenty of batty old women.

Still, scientists trip all over themselves trying to ensure that nobody places a value judgment on, say, the differences in brain size between the sexes. "Brain size should not be interpreted as implying any sort of functional advantage or disadvantage," tut-tutted the NIH-led team in the paper describing its work. Most scientists agree that the gap in manual dexterity between the genders has some in utero roots, but they hasten to add that later training amplifies the disparity, as more girls are taught to sew and more boys to shoot guns.

If the talents and aptitudes of the genders overlap, however, that's surely not how we start out. There is evidence that the brains of male and female fetuses begin diverging

even before genitals develop and hormones start pumping. Scientists have pinpointed one gene, for example, that seems to be responsible for the gender-based differences in motor skills, though so far that finding applies only to rats. Other studies have turned up 54 candidate genes that may play sex-differentiating roles in humans. "Plenty of the sex differences that happen in the mammalian brain happen by the time the mammal pops out of the womb," says Cahill. "While these differences tend to decrease with age as a general rule, they never disappear."

But why are they there in the first place? It seems not only unlikely but also wasteful that all these beefed-up brain parts would have made the evolutionary grade if they didn't provide some sort of significant advantage. After all, brains are biologically expensive. It can cost up to 10 times as much energy to keep a square centimeter of brain tissue running as it does an equivalent amount of any other organ. So any extra bulk had better be worth the energy—or at least have been worth it at some point in our evolution.

Hunting for just that sort of beneficial legacy, an international team of researchers published a paper in 1997 comparing differences in the brains of males and females of 21 species of primates—from highly social chimpanzees and gorillas to loners like rhesus monkeys. The researchers found that sociability is a great evolutionary force. While there were gender-based differences in the brains of all the species, those differences were much more obvious in the social primates than in the solitary ones.

Specifically, the parts of the brain in charge of aggression are much more substantial in males that live in groups—and must compete with other males for access to food and mates—than in their female counterparts. At the same time, the more competitive a male, the smaller his septum—the part of the brain that works to keep him levelheaded in a conflict—relative to that of females of his species and to less competitive males. That too makes sense: when it comes time to fight, rage trumps reason—at least sometimes.

In females, a larger group means a larger neocortex, the brain's cognitive center. If your job is to communicate with other females, figure out your place in the hierarchy and cooperate in gathering food and tending babies, your neocortex is just where you'd want a little extra heft.

Among humans, Cahill and his colleagues found that even when the brain is at rest, the right side of the amygdala, which processes emotionally influenced memories, is active in men, constantly communicating with other portions of the brain involved in external motor control—a way, perhaps, of staying on the alert for predators and other threats. In resting women, on the other hand, the left side is more active and connects with parts of the brain involved in the internal function of the body. This parallels the different ways pain is processed. Men's more analytic response to pain seems consistent with the traditional male role of planning a response to a threat, while women's more emotional response may be oriented more to protecting the brood.

Of course, evolutionary pressures don't, by themselves, shape brains. Some physiological process that translates survival needs into specialized brain tissue must play out. That process is driven by sex hormones—estrogens for women and testosterone for men.

"Circulating sex hormones are an absolutely crucial part of the story," says Cahill. "They are not, however, the entire story. There are plenty of examples of sex differences that exist independent of sex hormones." Indeed, the fact that scientists have been able to pinpoint gender differences in embryonic brains from developmental stages prior to the production of sex hormones proves that point.

"Even in adult animals that have lost their gonads, there are sex differences that remain," says UCLA neurophysiologist Arthur Arnold. "These are caused at least in part by the direct action of X and Y genes, which are present in different numbers in male and female cells."

The larger question, of course, is why these findings matter. It's hardly news, after all, that men and women are behaviorally different and that those differences must be brain-based. Still, one important lesson from the new science is that the brain is not destiny. Having a girl's language lobe or a boy's amygdala doesn't determine talents or temperament. It only suggests them.

"Experience matters," says Moore. "For instance, we can train people to do better on mental-rotation tests.

And we also know that baby boys and girls are treated differently right from birth, and that has an effect on brain development and behavior. So we need to consider that half of the story as well."

What's more, not every structural difference in the brain is significant; even in neuroscience, there are times when a cigar-shaped gyrus is just a cigar-shaped gyrus. Some differences in the structures of men's and women's brains may be no more relevant to how each sex functions than sex-linked traits like an Adam's apple or facial hair. Even the larger average size of men's brains—the most conspicuous difference—may be a result of nothing more than the larger average size of men's bodies.

More practically, what we discover about brain-based gender differences can teach us a lot about brain-based diseases. Many such ills—including Parkinson's disease, Tourette's syndrome and attention-deficit/hyperactivity disorder—are more prevalent in one sex than in the other, and the effectiveness of the treatments for those disorders may also have a gender bias. A 2008 study, for instance, found that women, while more prone to depression than men, were also one-third likelier to experience some relief of their symptoms when they took a particular antidepressant.

It may even be possible to take advantage of differences like this. "If we can find out what factor protects one sex from a disease that disproportionately affects the other," says Arnold, "we may be able to turn that factor into a drug that protects both sexes." And, he adds hopefully, we could do so reasonably safely. "Because most factors that cause sex differences are benign—after all, it wouldn't kill us to be the opposite sex—they may represent attractive candidates for drugs."

And for folks who prefer perfect equality of the sexes even when it comes to brains, take heart that many of the differences that remain may be fleeting—in evolutionary terms at least. We lost our tails and browridges and a lot more when we left the savanna. The more our gender roles overlap, the more the look and function of our brains may as well. Our bodies have always been works in progress; our brains will always be too. ∎

WHO'S BETTER AT WHAT?

Men	**Women**
BUILT FOR SIZE Male brains are 8% to 10% bigger and more densely packed with neurons	**ROOM TO NETWORK** Female brains have more space between neurons, which means more connections
POINT AND SHOOT Even correcting for cultural bias and training, male brains do better at target skills like archery and darts	**FINE CONTROL** Girls do better at skills like putting pegs in holes. Yes, this makes them good seamstresses— and also surgeons
MATH MUSCLE Boys excel at reasoning through a problem, but girls shine at straightforward tools like multiplication tables	**WORD POWER** Two key language centers are larger in females than in males, giving girls an edge in learning to talk
ON PATROL At rest, male brains stay active in areas that scan the world—perhaps looking for danger	**MINDING THE TRIBE** The left side of female brains stays more alert, overseeing internal and interpersonal matters

The Science Of Romance

Falling in love may be magical, but it's also chemical—a biological ride that starts in the brain but surely doesn't stop there

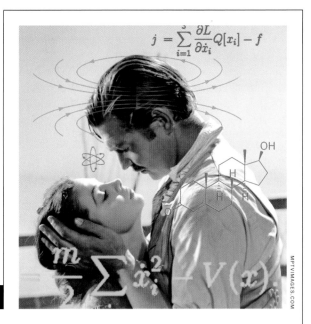

$$j = \sum_{i=1}^{3} \frac{\partial L}{\partial \dot{x}_i} Q[x_i] - f$$

$$\frac{m}{2} \sum \dot{x}_i^2 + V(x)$$

MPTVIMAGES.COM

THERE'S A LITTLE IRONY IN THE DIFFERing ways boys' and girls' brains develop. Because when all that maturing and specializing is done, the sexes are still expected to find sufficient common ground so that they can fall in love and spend the rest of their lives together. That's not easy when the ways they think, react and view the world are so dissimilar. Or it wouldn't be if the brain didn't have that covered too, simply by causing love to feel so good.

The earliest scans of brains in love were taken in 2000, and they revealed that the sensation of romance is processed in three regions. The first is the ventral tegmental area, a clump that is the body's central refinery for dopamine. Dopamine does a lot of jobs, but the thing we notice most is that it regulates reward. When you win a hand of poker, it's a dopamine jolt that's responsible for the thrill that follows. When you look forward to a big meal or expect a big raise, it's a steady flow of dopamine that makes the anticipation such a pleasure.

Helen Fisher, an anthropologist at Rutgers University, has conducted more-recent scans of people who are not just in love but newly in love and has found that their ventral tegmental areas are working particularly hard. "This little factory near the base of the brain is sending dopamine to higher regions," she says. "It creates craving, motivation, goal-oriented behavior—and ecstasy."

Even with its intoxicating supply of dopamine, the ventral tegmental area couldn't do the job on its own. Most people do leave the poker game or the dinner table, after all. Something has to turn the exhilaration of a new partner into what can approach an obsession. That something is the brain's nucleus accumbens, located slightly higher and farther forward. Thrill signals that start in the lower brain are processed in the nucleus accumbens via not just dopamine but also serotonin and, importantly, oxytocin, which is one of the chemicals that floods new mothers and creates such a fierce sense of connection to their babies.

"In one study, an aide who was not involved with the birth of a baby would stand in a hospital room while a mother was in labor," says Sue Carter, a professor of psychiatry at the University of Illinois. "The mothers later reported that they found the person very sympathetic, even though she was doing nothing at all." The same chemical put to work between lovers creates equally strong feelings.

The last major stops for love signals in the brain are the caudate nuclei, a pair of shrimp-size structures on either side of the head. It's here that patterns and mundane abilities such as knowing how to type or drive a car are stored. Motor skills like those can be hard to lose, thanks to the caudate nuclei's indelible memory. Apply the same permanence to love, and it's no wonder that passion can gel so quickly into commitment. The idea that even one part of the brain is involved in processing love would be enough to make the feeling powerful. The fact that three are at work makes that powerful feeling downright consuming. *—By Jeffrey Kluger*

POSTCARDS FROM THE BRAIN

The brain, wondrous as it is, poses a special challenge for scientists. Mental disorders play out in a 3-lb. universe that is largely inaccessible without extremely risky surgery. At least it was until the 1970s, when the first crude pictures of the living brain were taken. Today researchers can peer into that universe with a variety of technologies that capture the brain in action. The best results come from combining two or more scanning methods. Some capture the size and shape of brain structures; others freeze-frame the ever shifting activity of nerve cells as they fire and subside. With this information, doctors are beginning to understand—at the level of the neuron—how mental illnesses occur. Schizophrenia is the object of much of the pioneering work in this field, and many of the images on the following pages trace science's efforts to find the roots of the disorder—and perhaps someday a cure. —BY ALICE PARK

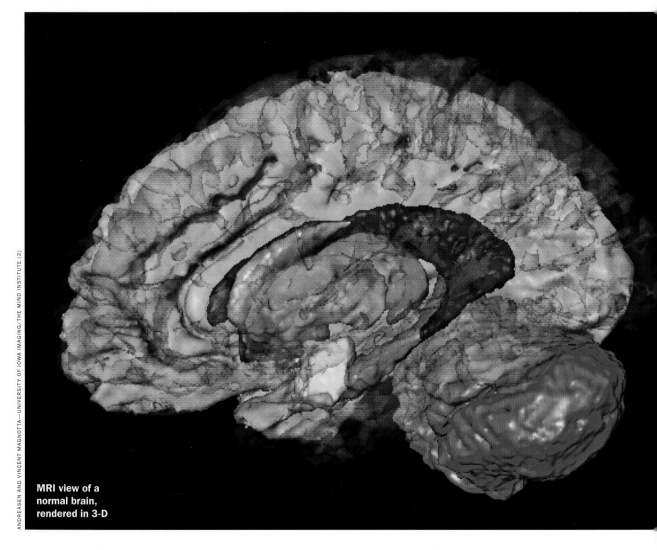

MRI view of a normal brain, rendered in 3-D

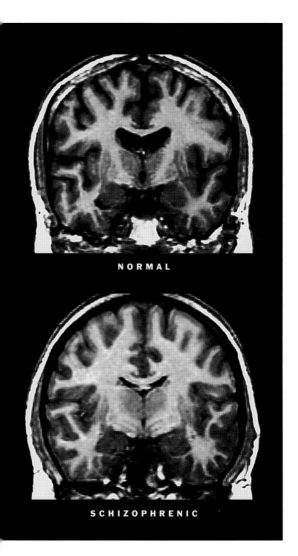

NORMAL   **SCHIZOPHRENIC**

NORMAL

SCHIZOPHRENIC

1970s
Computed Tomography (CT)

CT scans represent a major advance over the simple X-ray. Instead of a flat, two-dimensional picture, CT scanners produce a series of successive images. Taken as the patient, lying down, moves through a scanning ring, these "slices" can be combined to create the illusion of depth. The resulting pictures of bone and soft tissue can help doctors distinguish between patients with a psychiatric disorder and those with head trauma (which can trigger similar symptoms). CT scans have been particularly useful in identifying schizophrenia patients. In the 1970s, researchers for the first time uncovered a distinguishing abnormality in these patients' brains: the ventricles (fluid-filled spaces, circled in yellow, *left*), are significantly larger in those with the disease.

1980s
Magnetic Resonance Imaging (MRI)

This technology takes advantage of the body's natural magnetic field, measuring changes in the field's energy as patients are exposed to various radio frequencies. The system is particularly good at distinguishing among tissues of different densities. That is crucial in the case of soft tissues, which vary widely in composition and structure yet may all look the same to less discriminating imagers. Unlike CT views, MRIs can be rendered in true 3-D, because MRI machines can slice along three or more planes, not just one. A computer can then compile the information to generate a sort of relief map of the brain *(far left)* depicting even the smallest brain structures (for example, the brain's center for emotion, the amygdala, in yellow, is deeply buried but visible). Using MRIs, scientists have learned that the brains of schizophrenics *(left)* are smaller than those of people without the disease *(above left)* and have a smaller frontal lobe—the part of the brain responsible for planning, decision-making, higher learning and emotions. MRIs can also help diagnose tumors because the magnetic fields the scanner produces cause different kinds of protons in different types of tissue to line up and then return to their original positions at different rates.

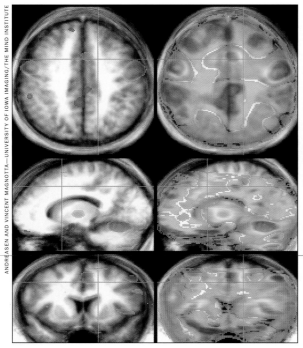

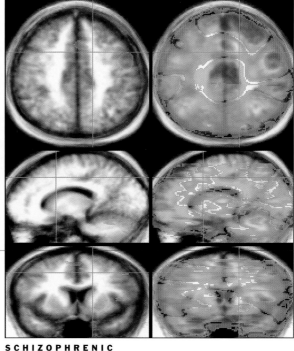

ANDREASEN AND VINCENT MAGNOTTA—UNIVERSITY OF IOWA IMAGING/THE MIND INSTITUTE

NORMAL **SCHIZOPHRENIC**

1980s

Positron-Emission Tomography (PET)

PET scans capture images of the brain in action. Patients receive an injection of a radioactive tracer that tracks how much blood is flowing through various regions and how much glucose is being broken down. PET images have proved indispensable for schizophrenia research, revealing that the disease stems from a difficulty distant brain regions have in communicating with one another. When schizophrenics are asked to remember words, the areas of the brain responsible for attention and working memory (in red, *above right*), activate at a lower level than in normal subjects *(above)*.

1990s

Functional Magnetic Resonance Imaging (fMRI)

An advance over PET imaging, fMRI measures brain function without radioactive tracers. Instead, it monitors how much oxygen brain cells are consuming. That serves as an indicator of how much blood is flowing to different regions, which in turn reveals how active nerve cells are. Typically fMRI subjects are placed in an MRI machine and asked to perform a mental task. Schizophrenic patients and normal subjects performing the same task activate the same brain regions (shown in yellow, *below*). But in schizophrenics, there is less blood flow, which indicates less nerve firing.

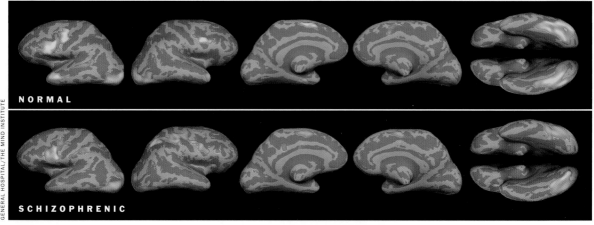

GINA KUPERBERG—MASSACHUSETTS
GENERAL HOSPITAL/THE MIND INSTITUTE

NORMAL

SCHIZOPHRENIC

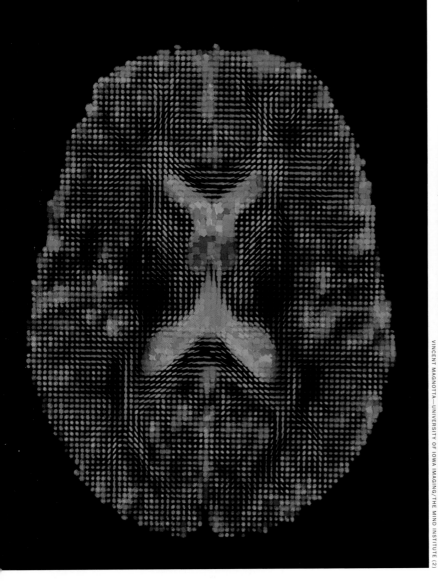

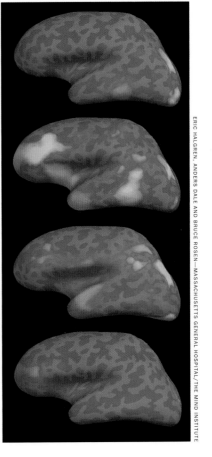

2000s

Diffusion Tensor Imaging (DTI)

As revealing as fMRI can be, no magnetic resonance image can accurately map the way different regions of the brain are wired together. That's because a lot of that wiring consists of fatty white matter, which does not appear in sharp definition on an MRI. DTI, however, looks specifically at the way water moves through white matter. Since the water flows along the strands of matter, following its route is like following the flow of a river—which yields a map of the riverbed beneath. In the large image *(top)*, the longer and narrower each discrete color dot, the sharper and more precise the track of the brain fibers. The data from such a scan can be analyzed to produce an image like the one in the smaller image *(above)*. This one focuses on the precise route and strength of individual strands—a bit like focusing on particular tributaries in a river valley. The U-shaped lines reveal an area of reduced connectivity in the frontal lobes of a schizophrenic, which may be responsible for the disease. DTI may have applications in diagnosing Alzheimer's disease and other types of dementia. It may also be used in diagnosing damage to skeletal and cardiac muscle.

Magneto-encephalography (MEG)

Not satisfied with just capturing images of the brain produced by such inferential clues as blood or water flow, scientists developed an exciting new technique that allows them to, in effect, directly see neurons fire. MEG does this by detecting changes in tiny magnetic signals produced by active neurons. This scan is ideal for tracing the order and pattern in which brain regions are activated when called upon to perform certain tasks. In this series of images *(above)*, a normal subject is presented with a list of new words to learn. The neurons fire in a wave that progresses from the back of the brain (in yellow, *above*), where the visual region is located, to the frontal lobes. Researchers are using the same technique with schizophrenic patients to learn whether there is a different pattern to their nerve firings. ■

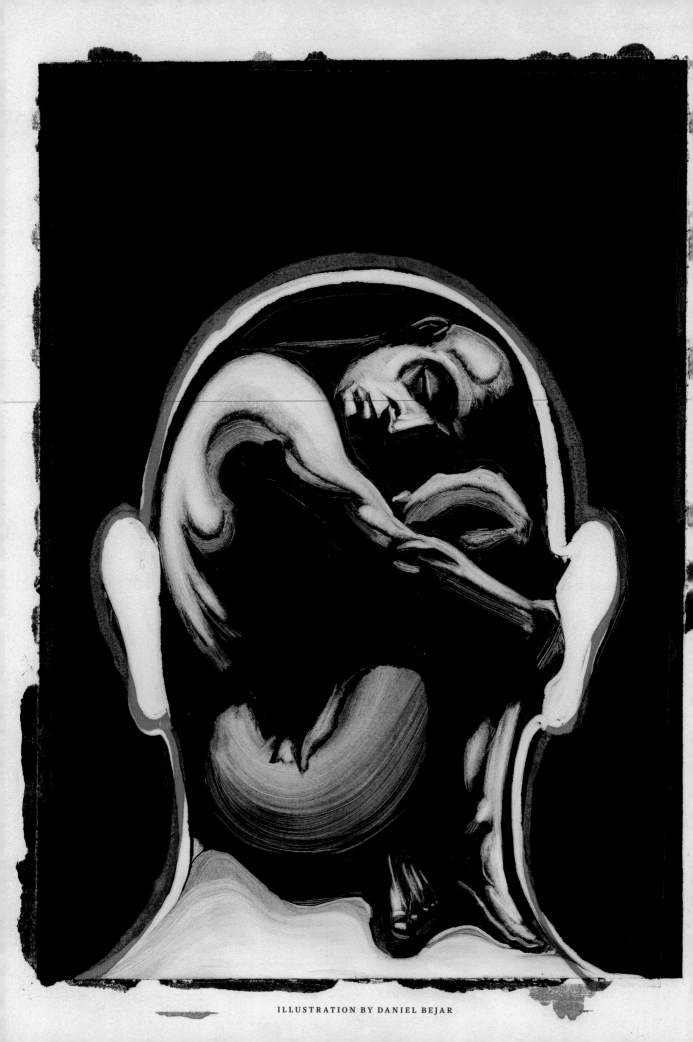

ILLUSTRATION BY DANIEL BEJAR

disorders

No machine as complex as the brain
can operate without malfunctions.
Illnesses of the mind have very real causes—and,
increasingly, very real treatments

Minds on The Edge

Imagine all your most powerful feelings welling up in you at once. Now imagine you can't resist acting on them. Welcome to borderline personality disorder

BY JOHN CLOUD

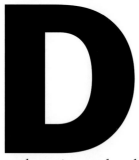

DOCTORS USED TO HAVE POetic names for diseases. A physician would speak of consumption because the illness seemed to eat you from within. Now we just use the name of the bacterium that causes the illness: tuberculosis. Psychology, though, remains a profession practiced partly as science and partly as linguistic art.

Because our knowledge of the mind's afflictions remains so limited, psychologists—even when writing in academic publications—still deploy metaphors to understand difficult disorders. And possibly the most difficult of all to fathom, and thus one of the most creatively named, is the mysterious-sounding borderline personality disorder (BPD). University of Washington psychologist Marsha Linehan, one of the world's leading experts on BPD, describes it this way: "Borderline individuals are the psychological equivalent of third-degree-burn patients. They simply have, so to speak, no emotional skin. Even the slightest touch or movement can create immense suffering."

And suffer they do. As many as 75% of BPD patients try to injure themselves, and approximately 10% commit suicide (by comparison, the suicide rate for mood

disorders is about 6%). Borderline patients seem to have no internal governor; they are capable of deep love and profound rage almost simultaneously. They are powerfully connected to the people close to them and terrified by the possibility of losing them—yet attack those people so unexpectedly that they often ensure the very abandonment they fear. When they want to hold, they claw instead.

A 2008 study of nearly 35,000 adults in the *Journal of Clinical Psychiatry* found that 5.9%—which would translate into 18 million Americans—had been given a BPD diagnosis. In contrast, clinicians diagnose bipolar disorder and schizophrenia in about 1% of the population. BPD has long been regarded as an illness disproportionately affecting women, but the latest research shows no difference in prevalence rates for men and women. Regardless of gender, people in their 20s are at higher risk for BPD than those older or younger.

What defines borderline personality disorder is the sufferers' inability to calibrate feelings and behavior. When faced with an event that makes them depressed or angry, they often become inconsolable or enraged. Such problems may be exacerbated by impulsive behaviors: overeating or substance abuse; suicide attempts; self-injury.

No one knows exactly what causes BPD, but the familiar nature-nurture combination of genetic and

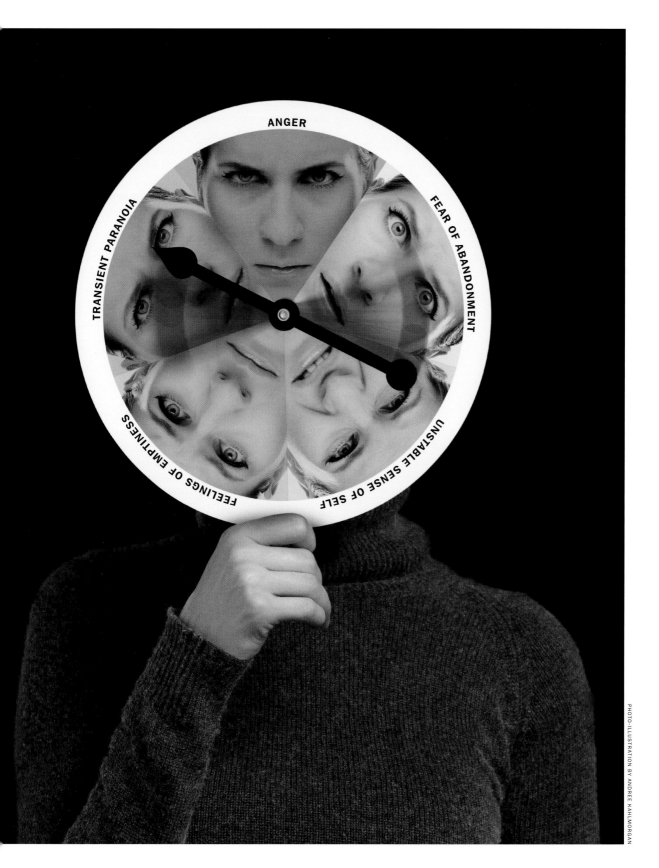

ANGER

FEAR OF ABANDONMENT

UNSTABLE SENSE OF SELF

FEELINGS OF EMPTINESS

TRANSIENT PARANOIA

Borderline patients are terrified of losing the people closest to them yet attack those people so unexpectedly that they often ensure the very abandonment they fear. When they want to hold, they claw instead

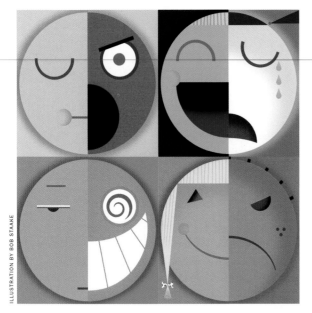

ILLUSTRATION BY BOB STAAKE

environmental misfortune is the likely culprit. There are several theories about why the number of borderline diagnoses may be rising. A parsimonious explanation is that because of advances in treating common mood problems like short-term depression, more health-care resources are available to identify difficult disorders like BPD. Another explanation is hopeful: BPD treatment has improved dramatically in the past few years. Until recently, a diagnosis of borderline personality disorder was seen as a "death sentence," as Dr. Kenneth Silk of the University of Michigan wrote in the April 2008 issue of the *American Journal of Psychiatry.* Clinicians often avoided naming the illness and instead told patients they had a less stigmatizing disorder.

Still, the rise in borderline diagnoses may illustrate something about our particular historical moment. Culturally speaking, many ages have their signature crack-up illness. In the 1950s, an era of postwar trauma, nuclear fear and the self-medicating three-martini lunch, it was anxiety. During the '60s and '70s, an age of suspi-

cion and Watergate, schizophrenics of the *One Flew over the Cuckoo's Nest* sort captured the imagination—mental patients as paranoid heroes.

So, is borderline the illness of our age? When so many of us are clawing to keep homes and paychecks, might we have become more sensitized to other kinds of desperation? In a world so uncertain, maybe it's natural to lose one's emotional skin. It's too soon to tell if that's the case, but BPD does have at least one thing in common with the recession. As Dr. Allen Frances, a former chair of the Duke University psychiatry department, has written, "Everyone talks about [BPD], but it usually seems that no one knows quite what to do about it."

But Linehan might. In the early 1990s, she became the first researcher to conduct a randomized study on the treatment of borderline personality disorder. The trial—which showed that a treatment she created, called dialectical behavior therapy, significantly reduced borderline patients' tendency to hurt themselves as well as the number of days they spent as inpatients—astonished the field.

Dialectical behavior therapy is so named because at its heart lies the requirement that both patients and therapists find synthesis in various contradictions, or dialectics. For instance, therapists must accept patients just as they are (angry, confrontational, hurting) within the context of trying to teach them how to change. Patients must end the borderline propensity for black-and-white thinking, while realizing that some behaviors are right and some are simply wrong.

"The patient's first dilemma," Linehan wrote in 1993's *Cognitive-Behavioral Treatment of Borderline Personality Disorder,* "has to do with whom to blame for her predicament. Is she evil, the cause of her own troubles? Or are other people in the environment or fate to blame? What the borderline individual seems unable to do is to hold both of these contradictory positions in mind."

Linehan's achievement was to realize that borderline patients are, in fact, on the borderline of many such dualities, and treatment must therefore be designed accordingly. Often that treatment is best described by a term that is itself a duality: tough love.

Among the most important techniques Linehan teaches her patients is one she calls the "wise mind"—a kind of calm, Zen state that she insists even the most debilitated patients can achieve. "Generally," she writes, "I have patients follow their breath … and try to let their focus settle into their physical center, at the bottom of their inhalation. That very centered point is wise mind." Another skill Linehan recommends is an anti-anger technique for social situations. "Don't make the situation worse," she counsels. "And, if possible, be a little tiny bit on the kind side. O.K.?"

What Is BPD?

It's a mental illness defined by the inability to regulate emotions. Patients must meet at least five of these nine criteria to receive a diagnosis of BPD

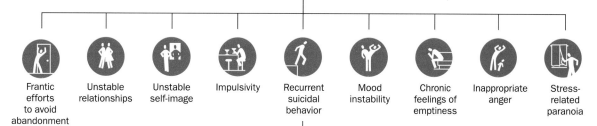

Frantic efforts to avoid abandonment · Unstable relationships · Unstable self-image · Impulsivity · Recurrent suicidal behavior · Mood instability · Chronic feelings of emptiness · Inappropriate anger · Stress-related paranoia

Why It's Dangerous

The combination of a mood disorder and an impulse-control problem *(see below)* confounds many therapists. Three in 4 BPD patients hurt themselves, usually by cutting or burning, and 1 in 10 commits suicide

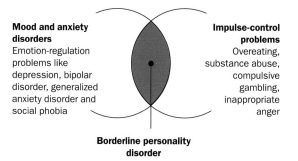

Mood and anxiety disorders
Emotion-regulation problems like depression, bipolar disorder, generalized anxiety disorder and social phobia

Impulse-control problems
Overeating, substance abuse, compulsive gambling, inappropriate anger

Borderline personality disorder

How It's Treated

The most widely studied treatment for BPD is called dialectical behavior therapy, which is designed to improve emotion regulation. How it works:

Individual therapy Helps patients identify stressors and feelings that precede self-injury and then teaches them how to stand apart from those feelings
Group therapy Patients learn skills like easing fear by engaging in social situations, not avoiding them
Case management Therapists consult with patients about how to interact with co-workers, health-care providers, family and friends
Drugs The literature provides little evidence that psychopharmaceuticals help people manage their BPD

The tough part of the tough love does not always go down so easily with patients. In *Cognitive-Behavioral Treatment of Borderline Personality Disorder,* for example, Linehan writes, "If the patient says, 'I am going to kill myself,' the therapist might reply, 'I thought you agreed not to drop out of therapy.'" In one intense session a few years ago, a patient told Linehan that her work stress was going to lead her to suicide. The patient said Linehan could never understand this stress because Linehan was a successful psychologist. Linehan responded, "I do understand. You can just imagine how stressful it is for me to have a patient constantly threatening to kill herself. Both of us have to worry about being fired!"

Such in-your-face tactics were highly controversial when Linehan started out. Other mental-health professionals publicly accused her of being heartless, even unethical. But her therapy has saved so many lives and worked so well in randomized trials that few criticize her today. Once, just after starting therapy with Linehan, a patient locked herself in her parents' bathroom and swallowed six or seven antidepressants in a half-hearted suicide attempt. The police were called, and they insisted the patient be taken to a hospital. Linehan advised the parents not to accompany her. She also told them they needed to make sure that the patient went to work the next day. The patient learned that she wouldn't be cosseted.

If some of this sounds like the stuff of kindergarten, it should. Remember that borderline patients have never learned to regulate their emotions. And just as teachers like to think there are no hopeless children, Linehan believes there are no hopeless patients. "Clients cannot fail," she says. "But both treatment and a therapist can fail."

Ever more therapists are willing to accept the challenge of treating BPD patients. Some 10,000 have been trained in dialectical behavior therapy, and more are signing on all the time. Even the best clinicians are unlikely ever to erase the psychic borderline that defines BPD—or even to define it precisely—but they can teach patients to be happy and healthy there. ∎

Through the Ages

You become susceptible to different disorders as your brain develops, matures and ages. Here's a guide to the typical age of onset

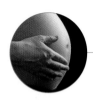

INFANCY TO BIRTH
Prenatal months

INFANCY
0 to 5 years old

LATE CHILDHOOD
5 to 10 years old

PUBERTY
10 to 13 years old

The brain and nervous system develop and form an intricate network. But genetic errors and environmental factors like fetal exposure to alcohol can make this process go awry. Some examples:

Excess neurons and synapses are pruned in the first 18 months, but the brain keeps growing, reaching 90% of adult size. Brain cells become more adept at communicating; babies learn to talk

Dramatic growth spurts in the temporal and parietal lobes, brain regions crucial to language and understanding of spatial relations, make this a prime time for learning new languages and music

Just before puberty, the brain's gray matter thickens, especially in the frontal lobe, the seat of planning, impulse control and reasoning. This growth may be triggered by surges of sex hormones

CEREBRAL PALSY
Affects about 10,000 U.S. babies a year. More than 80% show signs in the womb or before they are a month old. Usually diagnosed by age 3

FETAL ALCOHOL SYNDROME
Profound mental retardation caused by maternal alcohol abuse. Studies suggest that 1,200 to 8,800 FAS babies are born in the U.S. every year

NEURAL-TUBE DEFECTS
These include spina bifida and anencephaly, each of which affects 1 or 2 of every 10,000 live births

DOWN SYNDROME
The most common chromosome abnormality. Occurs in 1 of every 800 to 1,000 live births

TEXT BY
ANDREA DORFMAN

GRAPHIC BY
JACKSON DYKMAN

AUTISM DISORDERS
Three to four times as common in boys

EPILEPSY
About 10% of Americans will have a seizure sometime during their life. By age 80, about 3% will have been found to have epilepsy

DEPRESSION
In any given year, nearly 10% of adult Americans—two-thirds of them women—experience a depressive disorder. Up to 10% of children ages 6 to 12 have symptoms of major depression, but the typical age of onset is mid-20s

OBSESSIVE-COMPULSIVE DISORDER
Apparently caused by abnormally functioning brain circuitry. Neurotransmitter and hormone imbalances may also be involved

ANTISOCIAL BEHAVIOR
From lying and bullying to vandalism and homicide. More prevalent in boys, who tend to inflict physical harm on others

EATING DISORDERS
In the U.S., most common in teen girls and young women; only 5% to 15% of anorexics or bulimics and 35% of binge eaters are male

ATTENTION-DEFICIT/HYPERACTIVITY DISORDER
Tends to run in families and affects two to three times as many boys as girls. Between 3% and 5% of U.S. schoolchildren are thought to have ADHD

DYSLEXIA
Revealed when a child tries to learn to read

ANXIETY DISORDERS
Most prevalent group of psychiatric illnesses among children and adults

CONDUCT DISORDER
Various behaviors that show a persistent disregard for the norms and rules of society. Affects 6% to 16% of boys and 2% to 9% of girls under age 18

Sources: Dr. Jay Giedd, National Institute of Mental Health; Centers for Disease Control; National Center for Health Statistics; National Institute on Aging; National Institute of Child Health & Human Development; National Institute of Neurological Disorders and Stroke; MEDLINEplus; infoaging.org; American Psychiatric Association; American Academy of Child & Adolescent Psychiatry; MayoClinic.com; NAMI; National Mental Health Association

ADOLESCENCE
13 to 20 years old

The brain begins to shrink, losing about 2% of its weight and volume in each successive decade. Abnormally high loss of gray matter during this period may be a cause of teenage schizophrenia

EARLY ADULTHOOD
20 to 30 years old

By the late 20s, information processing begins to slow down. Memory centers in the hippocampus and frontal lobes seem most affected. This change is not usually noticeable until at least age 60

MIDDLE AGE
30 to 60 years old

Learning, memory, planning and other complex mental processes become more difficult, and reacting to stimuli takes longer. Plaques and tangles may form in certain brain regions

OLD AGE
60 to 100 years old

Aging, depression, anxiety disorders and Alzheimer's may alter sleep patterns. The decline in cognitive abilities becomes more pronounced. Coordination and dexterity are also affected

PANIC DISORDER

Afflicts 2.4 million Americans ages 18 to 54 in a given year. Twice as common in women

MENOPAUSE

Sudden mood swings, irritability, inability to cope, memory lapses

AGORAPHOBIA

Affects twice as many women as men

PARKINSON'S DISEASE

More than 1 million Americans have it

SOCIAL PHOBIAS

Persistent fears of being watched, judged or embarrassed in situations like parties or performing in public. Affect men and women equally

STROKE

Risk rises sharply after age 65

EARLY-ONSET ALZHEIMER'S

Just 5% to 10% of all Alzheimer's cases

ALZHEIMER'S DISEASE

Most common form of dementia among the elderly. Prevalence doubles every five years after age 65

POSTPARTUM DEPRESSION

Hits 10% of new mothers

PEAK SUICIDE YEARS

Third leading cause of death among people 15 to 24. White males are at greatest risk

HUNTINGTON'S DISEASE

More than 250,000 Americans have HD or are at risk of inheriting it

SCHIZOPHRENIA

Affects about 1% of the U.S. population

PEAK SUICIDE YEARS

People age 65 and older have higher suicide rates than any other age group. The rate among U.S. white men 85 and older is six times the national average

SEASONAL AFFECTIVE DISORDER

Most sufferers are women

BIPOLAR DISORDER

About 2.3 million adult Americans are manic-depressive

49

Pain, Rage And Blame

Personality disorders are among the toughest cases a psychologist can face. Other patients know they have a problem; these patients insist everybody else does

BY JEFFREY KLUGER

T HAS GOTTEN SO PSYCHOLOGIST LAWRENCE Josephs can tell right away which patients are likely to fire him—and it's usually the narcissists. These are the ones who are there in the first place only because their spouses would not quit hectoring them to show more interest in the marriage, or the people at work just didn't seem to give them the credit they deserve. Often, they stay only long enough to decide that what they really need is to leave the marriage or quit the job. After that, they sack the shrink.

"They come in under duress," says Josephs, a psychology professor at Adelphi University in Garden City, N.Y. "But what they really want is to have everything on their own terms."

If it's any comfort to Josephs, he's not alone in having such trouble with certain patients. Narcissism is one of 10 conditions under the diagnostic heading of personality disorders (PD), and patients with those conditions are among psychology's toughest nuts to crack. Talk therapy often doesn't touch them; drug therapy may do just as little. Disturbingly, as families increasingly fragment and societal pressures grow, experts say they are seeing more and more of these cases. As much as 9% of the population is thought to suffer from some kind of personality disorder, and as many as 20% of all mental-health hospitalizations may be a result of such conditions. "The more

severe [cases] are increasing," says Josephs, "especially among people who grew up in homes with divorce or drug and alcohol problems."

There are a lot of reasons personality disorders are so resistant to treatment, but the most important may be the way they insinuate themselves into the mind of the sufferer. Other mental conditions, such as anxiety disorders and depression, can be thought of as a pathological rind wrapped around an intact core. Peel the skin away through talk therapy or melt it away with drugs, and the problem may abate. Personality disorders, by contrast, are marbleized through the entire temperament. Narcissists may be self-absorbed, but they believe they jolly well have a right to be. "People rarely come in [to therapy] with a self-diagnosed personality disorder," says Josephs. "Friends and family push them."

These days they have more reason than ever to push. "The social costs of personality disorders are huge," says Dr. John Gunderson, director of the Personality Disorders Service at McLean Hospital in Belmont, Mass. "These people are involved in so many of society's ills—divorce, child abuse, violence. The problem is tremendous."

While solutions are elusive, the pathological arc of PDs is predictable. Symptoms tend to show up after age 18, striking men and women equally—though gender may influence which of the 10 disorders a person develops. The conditions are grouped into three sub-

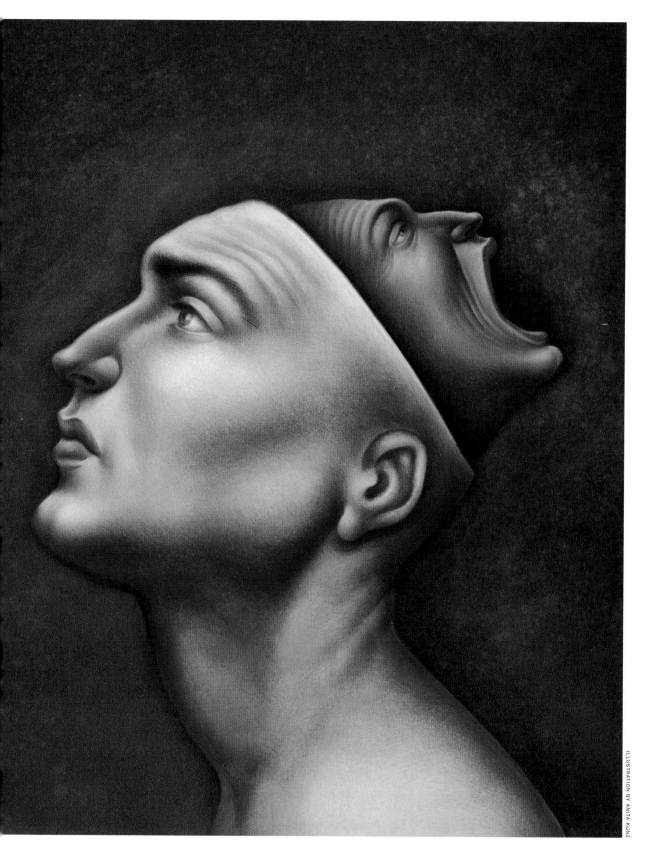

51

categories, and of these, the ones in the so-called dramatic cluster—borderline, antisocial, narcissistic and histrionic disorders—are the best known and the most explosive.

Less dramatic but just as stubborn is the so-called anxious cluster, including the straightforwardly named dependent personality, the socially withdrawn avoidant personality and the rigid and rule-bound obsessive-compulsive personality (a different diagnosis entirely from obsessive-compulsive disorder, an anxiety condition). The third group—actually called the odd cluster—includes the paranoid, schizotypal and schizoid personalities. Paranoid sounds like just what it is. Schizotypals and schizoids both have problems forming relationships and interpreting social cues. Schizotypals may also suffer delusions. "Schizoids are lone wolves," says Norman Clemens, a psychology professor at Case Western Reserve University in Cleveland. "Schizotypals skate along the edge of real schizophrenia."

Before scientists can figure out how to treat these conditions, they must first figure out what's behind them. Few researchers doubt that when disorders are so woven into temperament, some of what causes them is written into genes. A Norwegian study published in 2000 examined identical and fraternal twins and found that matched pairs—with their matched genetic blueprints—were more likely than unmatched pairs to share personality disorders. The borderline personality had an estimated 69% level of heritability.

But genes aren't everything. Therapists who work with narcissists often uncover childhood abuse or some other trauma leading to low self-esteem or even self-loathing—just the kind of emotional hole that pathological grandiosity would be designed to fill. Borderline-personality disorder affects more women than men, and some research has shown that up to 70% of borderline women were sexually or physically abused at some point in their lives. Poorly handled bipolar disorder or learning disabilities may also evolve into personality disorders.

Whatever the specific roots of the conditions, once those environmental and genetic dice are cast, is that it for the disordered personality? The short, bleak answer is often yes—at least as long as PD patients continue to resist acknowledging the problem. Anxiety disorders such as phobias are generally referred to as ego-dystonic illnesses: the sufferer knows that a problem exists and wants—sometimes deeply—to do something about it. Personality disorders are ego syntonic: individuals believe that the drama, self-absorption and other traits that characterize their condition are reasonable responses to the way the world is treating them. That's a hard patient to heal, but there is hope, and some of it starts in the pharmaceutical lab.

Researchers are finding that antipsychotics can help alleviate paranoid, schizoid and schizotypal symptoms. A variety of drugs—including mood stabilizers, anticonvulsants and SSRIs—may help control the impulsive element of the dramatic disorders. And while antidepressant and

DISORDERS

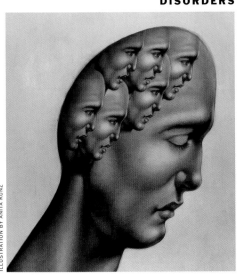

ILLUSTRATION BY ANITA KUNZ

Paranoid
A personality disorder that, as its name suggests, is characterized by suspicion and mistrust of others

Schizoid
Not schizophrenia; social isolation and limited range of emotional expression

Schizotypal
Not schizophrenia either, but getting dangerously close; similar to schizoid but with some delusions

Antisocial
Disregard of the law and the rights of others; a tendency toward deceit and manipulativeness

Borderline
Impulsiveness and volatility; a pattern of unstable relationships; often self-destructive or suicidal tendencies

Histrionic
Extreme emotionality and attention-seeking; may include excessive sexual seductiveness

Narcissistic
Grandiosity and self-absorption; an insatiable need for recognition; a lack of interest in others

Avoidant
A sense of inadequacy; extreme sensitivity to being seen as flawed; fear of social interaction

Dependent
Clinginess and submissiveness; difficulty assuming responsibility for decisions or disagreeing with others

Obsessive-Compulsive
Not OCD; similarly named personality disorder defined by rigidity and overadherence to rules

REWIRING THE BRAIN

In the summer of 2007, a 38-year-old man woke up and said hello to his mother. That ought not be news—except for the fact that the man had suffered severe brain damage in 1999 and spent eight years in the dark cognitive well known as a minimally conscious state.

The fact that the man is capable of any interaction is due to the therapeutic science of deep-brain stimulation (DBS). Doctors at the Cleveland Clinic inserted a pair of fine wires into his brain and threaded them down to the intact thalamus. Low current was sent through the wires, stimulating the thalamus, which awakened the higher brain.

Using DBS in severely brain-damaged patients is a brand-new breakthrough, but the technology has proved itself as a treatment for Parkinson's disease, is just beginning to be used for obsessive-compulsive disorder and is in clinical trials for depression. Studies suggest it could also help control symptoms of Alzheimer's disease, epilepsy and more. "DBS is like a pacemaker for the brain," says Cleveland Clinic neurosurgeon Ali Rezai, who performed the operation on the brain-damaged man. As with a pacemaker, the battery pack and charging unit for the system are implanted under the skin of the chest.

The Cleveland Clinic is one of 250 places in the U.S. that perform DBS for Parkinson's, and, worldwide, close to 40,000 people have undergone the procedure. But the operation is not a cure. For one thing, it doesn't do much for end-stage Parkinson's symptoms. More important, Parkinson's is a degenerative condition, which means that while DBS neutralizes tremors, the brain continues to deteriorate. After a decade or so, electrical stimulation is not enough. Still, that's 10 relatively symptom-free years during which other treatments may become available.

The benefits of DBS would have a similar expiration date for a disease like Alzheimer's, but in the case of anxiety or mood disorders, it could approach a true cure. A broken brain, in effect, would be fixed. —*J.K.*

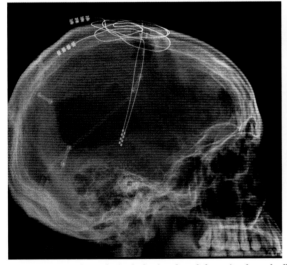
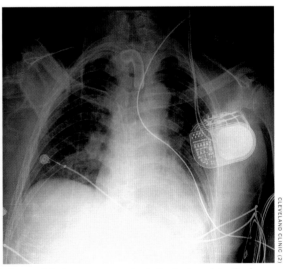

CLEVELAND CLINIC (2)

Mind boosters *Electrodes in the brain, above left, restimulate a badly damaged thalamus; a pacemaker in the chest regulates the charge*

antianxiety medications do little to rejigger something as fundamental as personality, doctors find that if they prescribe the drugs to relieve the stress that comes with living so disordered a life, some motivated patients may then take on the harder work of talk therapy.

For those who do, the options are growing. Cognitive and behavioral therapy in particular can teach coping skills, helping people get a more honest view of their lives and then fix what's not working. A study conducted by Gunderson and colleagues at Harvard, Yale, Columbia and Brown looked at borderline, avoidant, obsessive-compulsive and schizotypal patients and found that after two years of treatments, they showed a 40% improvement. "That's big news," says Gunderson. "Nobody would have thought we'd get better than 15%."

Forty percent, however, still leaves 60% suffering, and researchers are working to tip that balance the other way. Until they do, it will mostly be up to patients to deny the lie that the disorder tells—that there's really nothing wrong with them—and make the therapeutic commitment necessary to get well. "Nobody totally changes," says Josephs. "But anyone can become more flexible and resilient. Anyone can make progress." That alone is already a better prognosis than most patients have had. ■

Medicine Chest for the Mind

A pill can't make you happy, but a growing collection of drugs may at least ease the way

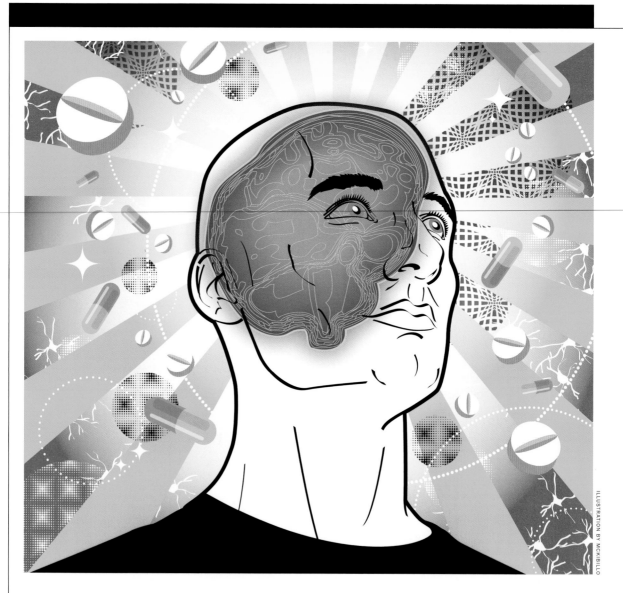

THERE IS NO ANTIBIOTIC FOR MADNESS, NO analgesic for psychic pain. The disorders that torment the mind are not caused by something as singular as a bacterium or a virus. That, however, has not kept humans from hunting for peace in a pill—or a poultice or root or leaf or fungus.

It's been thousands of years since we first discovered that the complicated chemistry that governs our brains can be radically altered by a little extra chemistry we drink or smoke or chew. We learned of the visions hidden in the peyote cactus, the vigor that could come from the coca leaf. There was lethal bliss in the pod of the poppy, sloppy fun in fermenting fruit, a jittery kick in the simple coffee bean. Still other kinds of pleasure were found in the cannabis plant, the psilocybin mushroom and more.

A natural pharmacopoeia like this and a creative brain like ours made it a certainty that we'd find better and better ways to make use of such intoxicating chemistry—often disastrously, but sometimes curatively. Physicians and psychiatrists—to say nothing of patients suffering from psychic disorders—have long searched for pharmacological ways to ease emotional suffering, even if that suffering could never be medicated away entirely. In the Victorian era, the drug of choice was laudanum, a high-octane mix of ethanol and opium that packed just the chemical wallop it sounds it would. The drug was used as a painkiller, an antidepressant and an antihysteric, and it often worked quite well—provided you overlooked the fact that it was also wildly addictive and frequently lethal.

In the late 19th and early 20th centuries, lithium was the hot new thing. A chemical salt derived from an alkali metal, lithium did not provide the intoxication laudanum did and was used mostly to ease the manic cycles suffered by patients with bipolar disorder. In the 1950s, the so-called tricyclics became popular. Named after their three-ring molecular structure, tricyclics helped block the reabsorption of neurotransmitters in the brain and alleviate symptoms of depression. Both kinds of drugs, however, were blunt instruments, with sometimes unbearable side effects like thirst, weight gain, lethargy and memory impairment.

Still, the drug train roared on, with antipsychotics like Thorazine, for schizophrenia; depressants like Valium, for anxiety; stimulants like Ritalin, for attention-deficit/hyperactivity disorder; and selective serotonin reuptake inhibitors like Prozac, for depression.

All these drugs have been refined over the years, and all have spawned subtler, more precisely targeted formulations that work better and cause fewer side effects. All too have given rise to worries that we're in danger of becoming too dependent on our chemical crutches, unable to buck up and get through tough times without relying on a pill to make a worry go away. But carefully prescribed and judiciously used, medication for the mind—just like medication for the body—not only can improve lives but also can save them. The trick is understanding just what medicines are out there and just when it's wise to avail yourself of the help they offer. —*By Jeffrey Kluger*

DRUG TYPES	WHAT THEY TREAT	HOW THEY WORK	SIDE EFFECTS
ANTIDEPRESSANTS Prozac, Paxil, Celexa, Zoloft, Lexapro, Effexor, Wellbutrin, Anafrinil, Elavil	The term *antidepressant* is a bit misleading because the drugs are also used to treat obsessions, compulsions and general anxiety	Most work by blocking the reabsorption of serotonin. Anafrinil and Elavil are tricyclics, which work similarly but with worse side effects	Fatigue, weight gain, reduced libido, thirst, disruption of sleep, suicidal thoughts. Quitting the drugs must be done gradually
SEDATIVES Valium, Xanax, Klonopin, Librium, Nembutal, Seconal, Ativan, Tranxene	Used for treating sleeplessness, anxiety, stress, pain and panic, sedatives can be extremely effective but also exceedingly addictive	Two main types: barbiturates and benzodiazepines. Both boost the neurotransmitter GABA, which slows the central nervous system	Addiction is the main risk—and it's a big one. Overdoses (accidental or not) are common, particularly when alcohol is consumed too
STIMULANTS Dexedrine, Ritalin, Strattera, Attenta, Preludin, Sanorex, Provigil, Fastin and, of course, caffeine	Narcolepsy, attention-deficit/hyperactivity disorder (most commonly in children), obesity, fatigue, sometimes depression	Increase norepinephrine and dopamine in the brain; also trigger release of these chemicals from storage areas in cells	Addiction, chest pains and other cardiac symptoms, impulsiveness, mood swings, insomnia, anorexic weight loss, delusions
ANTIPSYCHOTICS Haldol, Loxitane, Thorazine, Prolixin, Serentil, Risperdal, Seroquel, Zyprexa	Symptoms of psychoses, including hallucinations and agitation. Newer atypical antipsychotics treat bipolar disorder as well	Block dopamine receptors in brain pathways, though not always very selectively. Atypical formulations also block serotonin receptors	Numerous, including involuntary muscle movements, weight gain, cardiac symptoms, seizures, lethargy, low blood pressure
MOOD STABILIZERS Lithium, Lamotrigine, Lamictal, Depakote, Tegretol, Neurontin, Topamax	Generally used to treat the highs and lows of bipolar disorder, though not all the drugs in this class are FDA-approved for that use	Two types: anticonvulsants, originally used for epilepsy, mediate GABA function. The mechanism of lithium, the other main class, is unclear	Tremors, weight gain, headaches, sleepiness, rashes, vomiting, dizziness, liver toxicity, abnormal blood counts

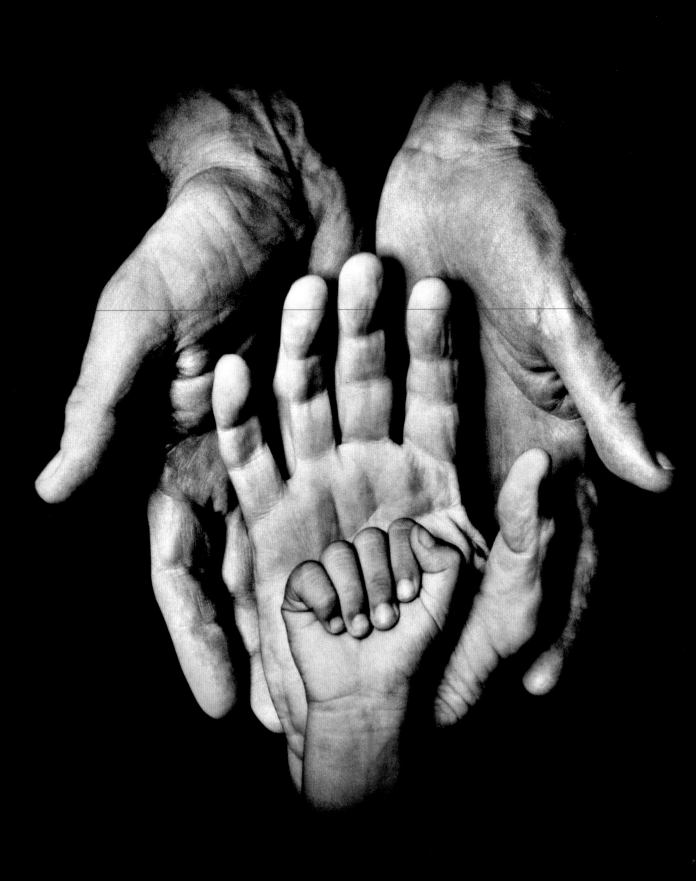

maturing

You're born with a brain that pulses with potential. It begins to
learn with your first breath—and doesn't stop until your last

Gray Hair And Wise Brains

You might be more forgetful than you
used to be, but the mind you have in your
later decades may be subtler, nimbler
and flat-out smarter than it's ever been

BY JEFFREY KLUGER

T TOOK BARBARA HUSTEDT CROOK AN AW-
fully long time to get around to writing her first
musical. She started shortly before her 60th
birthday. Her friend and collaborator, Robert
Strozier, waited even longer—until he turned 65.
It's not that they didn't have the creative chops
for the job. The two have spent their careers as
full-time writers and editors, and Crook has a
background in performing, singing and piano-
playing. But creating a musical always felt just
out of reach—until they arrived in their seventh decades.

"Somehow I have a confidence I didn't have before,"
says Crook. "I find that my brain makes leaps it didn't
make so easily." And, says Strozier, they're both a lot
more willing to take chances. "At a certain age," he says,
"you either get older or you get younger. If you get younger, you venture out and take risks."

Risk-taking seniors making daring mental leaps?
That's not the stereotype. Until quite recently, researchers believed the human brain followed a predictable arc.
It started out protean, gained shape and intellectual muscle as it matured, and reached its peak by age 40. After
that, it began a slow decline, clouding up bit by bit until,
by 60 or 70, it had lost much of its ability to retain new
information and fumbled with what it did know.

That, as it turns out, is hooey. More and more, neurologists and psychologists are coming to the conclusion that
the brain at midlife—a period increasingly defined as the
years from 35 to 65 and even beyond—is much more elastic
than anyone realized.

Far from slowly powering down, the brain begins
bringing new cognitive systems online and cross-indexing
existing ones in ways it never did before. You may not be
able to pack as much raw data into your memory as you
could when you were in college, and your short-term memory may not be what it was, but you manage information
and parse meanings that were beyond you when you were
younger. What's more, your temperament changes to suit
those new skills, growing more comfortable with ambiguity and less susceptible to frustration or irritation.

"In midlife," says UCLA neurologist George Bartzokis,
"you're beginning to maximize the ability to use the en-
tirety of the information in your brain on a second-to-
second basis. Biologically, that's what wisdom is."

If your mind does indeed grow more agile as you age,
one of the things that may help it do so is the amount of
glue—or glia, the Greek word that anatomists use—you
carry around in your brain. Only about half the mass of
the brain is composed of gray matter—actual nerve cells.
The rest is white matter, the connecting tissue that, in a
sense, glues it all together. Much of that white matter is
made of conductive nerve strands, and covering each fine
wire is a fatty sheath of myelin that keeps nerve signals
from sputtering out or cross-firing during transmission.

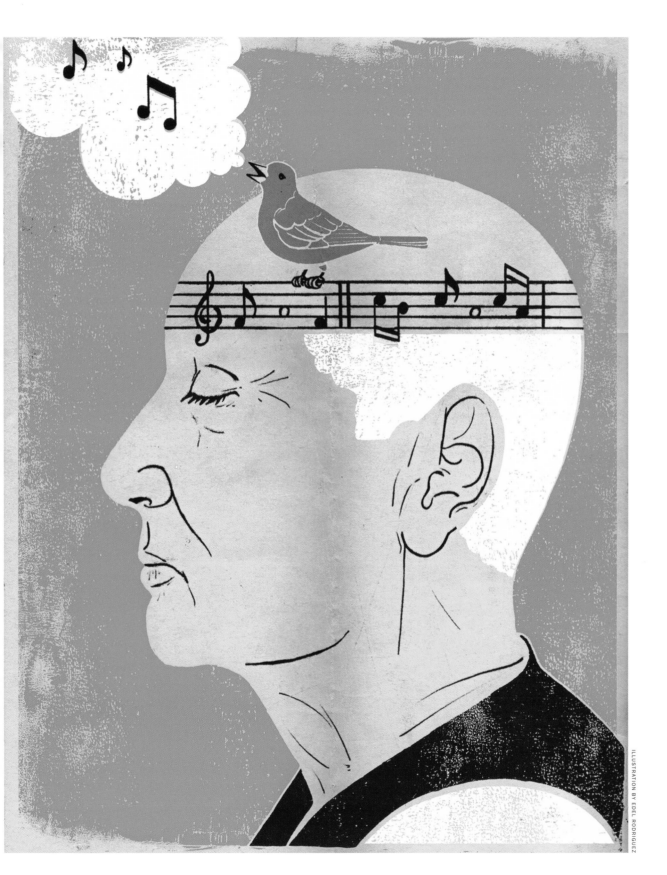

Throughout our lives, fresh layers of myelin sheathing are laid down in the brain. In infants and children, the bulk of it forms in the motor and sensory lobes. If we acquire better reasoning skills in middle age, Bartzokis long suspected, it would follow that most of the myelin added in those years would appear around the signal-transmitting axons in the higher brain regions that are the seat of sophisticated thought.

To test that idea, Bartzokis used magnetic resonance imaging (MRI) to study the volume and distribution of white matter in 300 healthy subjects from 18 to 75 years old as well as in hundreds of older people suffering

Older Can Be Better

As befits so complex an organ, the brain ages in numerous ways. Some of its abilities decline with the years, but others keep improving with use

from such brain-related ills as Alzheimer's disease. As he suspected, the healthy adults had more myelin in the frontal and temporal lobes—where big thoughts live. The quantity of sheathing reached its peak at around 45 or 50, exceeding the amount in unhealthy older subjects as well as healthy younger ones. "This last little bit of myelination essentially puts us online," Bartzokis says.

It's not just the wiring that charges up the brain as we age; it's the way different regions start pulling together. The brain's left and right hemispheres often work almost independently of each other. One hemisphere can be busy writing a grocery list or solving an equation while the other scans the environment and tends to basic chores. As we age, however, the walls between the hemispheres seem to fall.

To demonstrate that, neuroscientist Roberto Cabeza of Duke University recruited a sample group of adults from 65 to 95 years old who had scored high on a memory test, along with a group of lower-performing adults of the same age and a group of college-age adults. He asked them all to perform a series of cognitive tasks and conducted functional MRI scans of their brains as

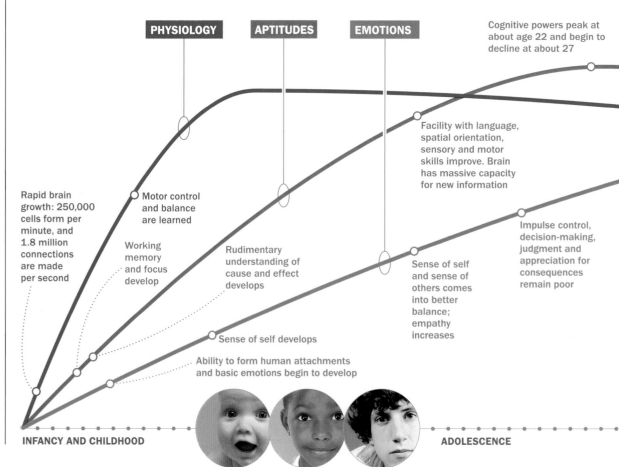

PHYSIOLOGY   **APTITUDES**   **EMOTIONS**

Cognitive powers peak at about age 22 and begin to decline at about 27

Facility with language, spatial orientation, sensory and motor skills improve. Brain has massive capacity for new information

Rapid brain growth: 250,000 cells form per minute, and 1.8 million connections are made per second

Motor control and balance are learned

Impulse control, decision-making, judgment and appreciation for consequences remain poor

Working memory and focus develop

Rudimentary understanding of cause and effect develops

Sense of self and sense of others comes into better balance; empathy increases

Sense of self develops

Ability to form human attachments and basic emotions begin to develop

INFANCY AND CHILDHOOD   **ADOLESCENCE**

they worked. Again and again, he found that the high-functioning older adults were either using a different hemisphere from that employed by the other subjects or using both at the same time.

Cabeza believes that while the brain does get weaker as it ages, each hemisphere compensates for this decline by outsourcing some of its work to the other, often integrating their efforts so smoothly that your reasoning is actually better than it was before. "It's similar to the way you need both hands to lift a weight that you could lift with one hand when you were younger," Cabeza says.

As the brain's flexibility improves, so too may temperament. In 1958, psychologist Ravenna Helson, now a professor emeritus at the University of California, Berkeley, began a long-term study of 142 women at Mills College in nearby Oakland. She interviewed the subjects and took measures of their personalities, drives, relationship skills and the like. Then she reinterviewed them at ages 27, 43, 52 and 61 to determine how those traits changed over time. In 2005, she and a graduate student, psychologist Christopher Soto, collated the data from the 123 women who had remained in the study.

On the whole, the women's highest scores in inductive reasoning, equanimity and objectivity occurred from their 40s to their early 60s. There was also an increased tolerance for ambiguity and an improved ability to manage relationships. This, says psychologist Robert Levenson, also at U.C. Berkeley, may be shaped in part by evolution. Human beings' long life spans and extended families are good things, but keeping big broods healthy and well behaved over the decades requires more than the energy of young parents. It takes the cool heads and wise counsel of the family graybeards too. "Evolution isn't just about reproduction," Levenson says. "When you get into your 40s and 50s, you're caretaking, looking after your children, grandchildren, the people who work for you."

It's that talent for reflective thinking that explains the role older adults have always played in human culture. It's not for nothing that history's firebrands and ideologues are typically young, while its judges and peacemakers and great theologians tend to be older. Not everyone achieves the sharp thought and serene mien that can come with age. But for those who do, the later years can be the best they have ever had. ■

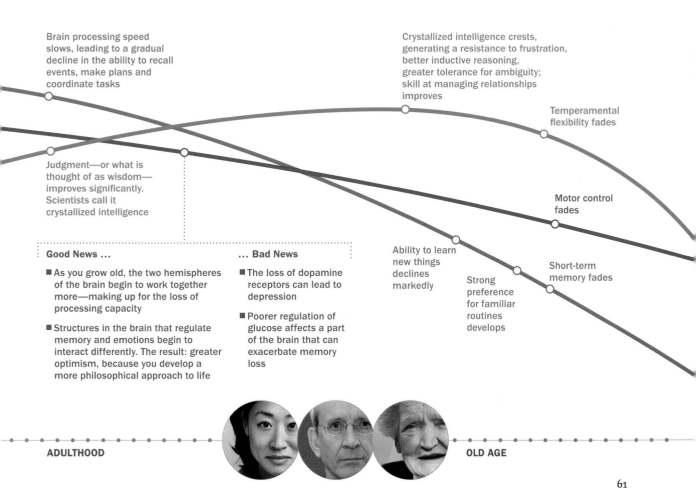

Brain processing speed slows, leading to a gradual decline in the ability to recall events, make plans and coordinate tasks

Crystallized intelligence crests, generating a resistance to frustration, better inductive reasoning, greater tolerance for ambiguity; skill at managing relationships improves

Temperamental flexibility fades

Judgment—or what is thought of as wisdom—improves significantly. Scientists call it crystallized intelligence

Motor control fades

Good News ...

■ As you grow old, the two hemispheres of the brain begin to work together more—making up for the loss of processing capacity

■ Structures in the brain that regulate memory and emotions begin to interact differently. The result: greater optimism, because you develop a more philosophical approach to life

... Bad News

■ The loss of dopamine receptors can lead to depression

■ Poorer regulation of glucose affects a part of the brain that can exacerbate memory loss

Ability to learn new things declines markedly

Strong preference for familiar routines develops

Short-term memory fades

ADULTHOOD

OLD AGE

The Wild World of a Teen Brain

Adolescence can be a volatile time, but the storms that play out in the home are nothing compared with what's going on in the heads of the teens themselves

BY CLAUDIA WALLIS

FIVE YOUNG MEN IN SNEAKERS and jeans troop into a waiting room at the National Institutes of Health Clinical Center in Bethesda, Md., and drape themselves all over the chairs in classic collapsed-teenager mode. It's midafternoon, and they are, of course, tired, but their presence adds a jangly, hormonal buzz to the bland, institutional setting. The teens are here to have their heads examined. Literally. They are participants in a giant study that's been going on in this building since 1991. Its goal: to determine how the brain develops from childhood into adolescence and on into early adulthood.

It is the project of Dr. Jay Giedd, chief of brain-imaging in the child-psychiatry branch at the National Institute of Mental Health. Giedd uses magnetic resonance imaging (MRI) to peek at kids' brains over the years and find physiological changes that might account for the adolescent behaviors so familiar to parents: emotional outbursts, recklessness, rule-breaking and the impassioned pursuit of sex, drugs and rock 'n' roll.

One reason scientists have been so intrigued by the ferment in the teenage brain is that the brain grows very little over the course of childhood. By the time a child is 6, the brain is 90% to 95% of its adult size. As a matter of fact, we are born equipped with most of the neurons our brain will ever have—and that's fewer than we have in utero. What Giedd's long-term studies are documenting is that there is a second wave of neuron proliferation and pruning that happens later in childhood and that the final, critical part of this second wave, affecting some of our highest mental functions, occurs in the late teens.

No matter how a particular brain turns out, its development proceeds in stages, generally from back to front. Some of the regions that reach maturity earliest are those in the back of the brain that mediate direct contact with the environment by controlling such sensory functions as vision, hearing, touch and spatial processing. Next are areas that coordinate those functions. The very last part of the brain to be shaped to its adult dimensions is the prefrontal cortex, home of the so-called executive functions—planning, prioritizing, organizing thoughts, suppressing impulses, weighing consequences.

"Scientists attributed the bad decisions teens make to hormones," says Elizabeth Sowell, a UCLA neuroscientist who has done seminal MRI work on the developing brain. "But once we started mapping brain changes, we could say, Aha, the part of the brain that makes teenagers more responsible is not finished maturing."

Hormones, however, do remain an important part of the teen-brain story. At puberty, the ovaries and testes

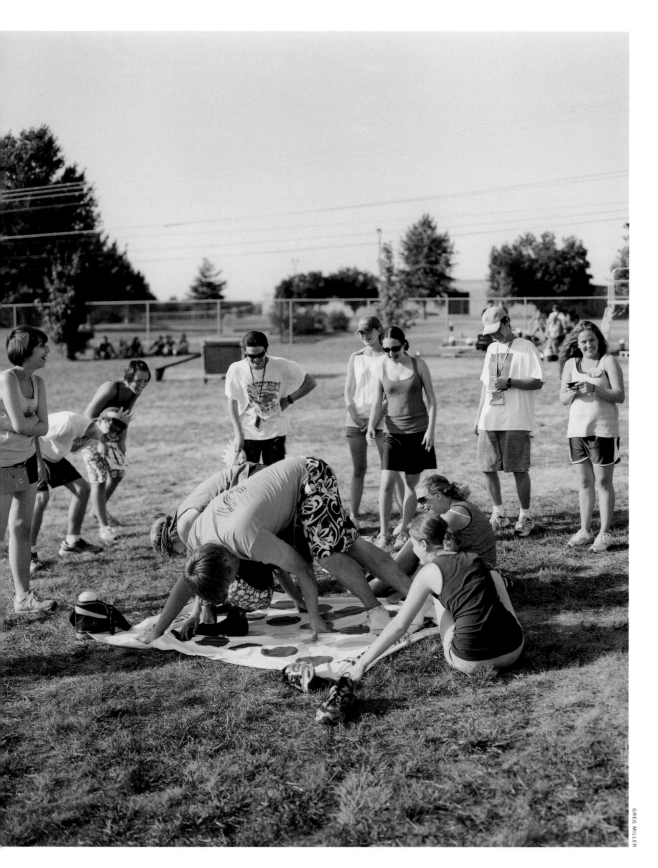

63

begin to pour estrogen and testosterone into the bloodstream. At the same time, testosterone-like hormones released by the adrenal glands, located near the kidneys, begin to circulate. Recent discoveries show that these hormones are extremely active in the brain, especially in the emotional center—the limbic system. This creates a "tinderbox of emotions," says Dr. Ronald Dahl, a psychiatrist at the University of Pittsburgh. Not only do feelings reach a flash point more easily, but adolescents also tend to seek out situations that allow their emotions and passions to run wild. "Adolescents are actively looking for experiences to create intense feelings," says Dahl.

Psychologists are investigating the brain to explain other kinds of wacky adolescent behavior. At McLean Hospital in Belmont, Mass., Harvard neuropsychologist Deborah Yurgelun-Todd did an elegant series of functional MRI experiments in which both kids and adults were asked to identify the emotions displayed in photographs of faces. "In doing these tasks," she says, "kids and young adolescents rely heavily on the amygdala, a structure in the temporal lobes associated with emotional reactions. Adults rely less on the amygdala and more on the frontal lobe."

And what about why it's so hard to get a teenager off the couch? You might blame that on an immature nucleus accumbens, a brain region that directs motivation to seek rewards. James Bjork at the National Institute on Alcohol Abuse and Alcoholism used brain scans to study motivation in a challenging gambling game. He found that teenagers have less activity in this region than adults do. "If adolescents have a motivational deficit, it may mean that they are prone to engaging in behaviors that have either a really high excitement factor or a really low effort factor, or both," he says. Sound familiar?

In light of what's being learned, it seems almost arbitrary that our culture has decided that a young American is ready to drive a car at 16, vote and serve in the military at 18 and drink alcohol at 21. Giedd says the best estimate for when the brain is truly mature is 25. Some legal scholars and children's advocates also argue that minors should never be tried as adults and should be spared the death penalty. In 2003 the American Bar Association urged all state legislatures to ban the death penalty for juveniles "for social and biological reasons."

Most parents, of course, know instinctively about the limited nature of the teen brain. What bears remembering is that there's only so much even the best child-rearing practices can do about it. "You can tell [teens] to shape up or ship out," Giedd says, "but making mistakes is part of how the brain grows." It might be more useful for parents to help kids make up for what the brain still lacks by providing structure and guidance and applying those time-tested virtues: patience and love. ∎

Inside the Adolescent Brain

The brain undergoes two major developmental phases, one in the womb and a second that takes place from childhood through the teen years. The maturation occurs in a predictable pattern, spreading from the back of the brain to the front

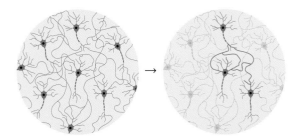

Nerve Proliferation and Pruning

By age 11 for girls and 12½ for boys, the neurons in the front of the brain have formed thousands of new connections. Over the next few years, many of these links will be pruned. Those that are used and reinforced—the pathways involved in language, for example—will be strengthened, while the ones that aren't used will die out

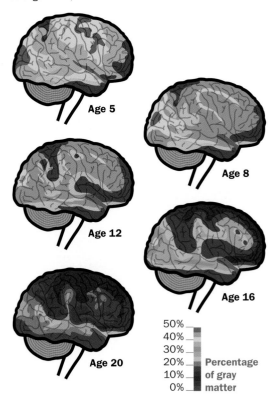

Age 5

Age 8

Age 12

Age 16

Age 20

50%
40%
30%
20% — Percentage
10% — of gray
0% — matter

Time-Lapse Brain

Gray matter wanes as the brain matures. Here, 15 years of brain development are compressed into five images showing a shift from red (least mature) to purple (most mature)

Sources: Dr. Jay Giedd, chief of brain-imaging, child-psychiatry branch, NIMH; Paul Thompson, Andrew Lee, Kiralee Hayashi and Arthur Toga, UCLA Lab of Neuro Imaging; Nitin Gogtay and Judy Rapoport, child-psychiatry branch, NIMH. Text by Kristina Dell

GRAPHIC BY ROBERT A. DI IESO JR.

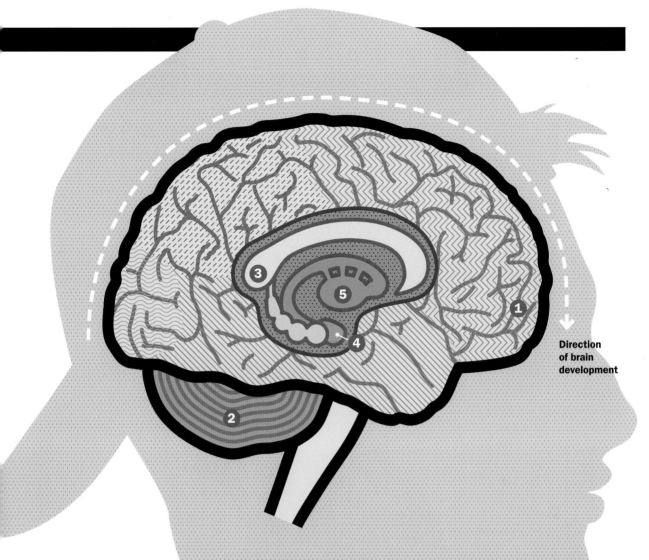

Direction of brain development

1. Prefrontal Cortex

The CEO of the brain, also called the area of sober second thought, is the last part of the brain to mature—which may be why teens get into so much trouble. Located just behind the forehead, the prefrontal cortex grows during the preteen years and then shrinks as neural connections are pruned during adolescence.

2. Cerebellum

Long thought to play a role in physical coordination, this area may also regulate certain thought processes. More sensitive to the environment than to heredity, the cerebellum supports activities of higher learning like mathematics, music and advanced social skills. New research shows that it changes dramatically during adolescence.

3. Corpus Callosum

Thought to be involved in problem-solving and creativity, this bundle of nerve fibers connects the left and right hemispheres of the brain. During adolescence, the nerve fibers thicken and process information more and more efficiently.

4. Amygdala

This region is the emotional center of the brain, home to such primal feelings as fear and rage. When they are processing emotional information, teens tend to rely more heavily on the amygdala, whereas adults depend more on the rational prefrontal cortex, which is under-developed in teens. The impulsive decisions, arguments and door slams of the adolescent are the amygdala at work.

5. Basal Ganglia

Larger in females than in males, this part of the brain acts like a manager for the prefrontal cortex by helping it prioritize information. The basal ganglia and prefrontal cortex are tightly connected: at nearly the same time, they both grow and prune neuronal connections. This area is also active in directing and coordinating small and large motor movements, so it may be important to expose preteens to music and sports while it is growing.

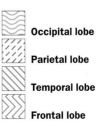

Occipital lobe

Parietal lobe

Temporal lobe

Frontal lobe

THE FACES OF GENIUS

There is perhaps no other word that's been so cheapened by overuse as *genius*. Was Einstein a genius? Sure. Mozart? Definitely. What about Yo-Yo Ma? Jonas Salk? Tiger Woods? What about the mother who looks at a child and intuits instantly its needs and feelings? Isn't that a powerful form of genius too? Perhaps the truest measure of genius is what it does. If that's so, the gallery that follows is made of geniuses indeed

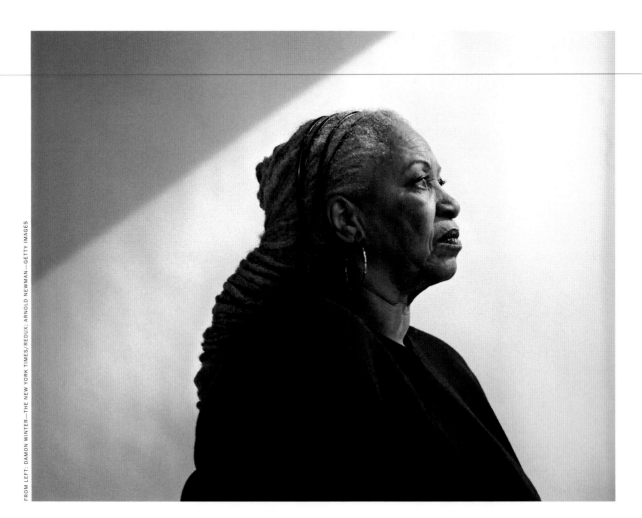

TONI MORRISON

Yes, there's the Nobel, and, yes, there's the Pulitzer, and Morrison, above, has them both on her shelves. But the true prizes are her words, and they're not honors she receives but gifts she gives. "You your best thing," one of her characters says to another in her landmark book *Beloved*. Morrison's writing, in turn, is one of American literature's best things

PABLO PICASSO

Never has the arc of an artist's work so matched the arc of his era. Wars and upheaval fractured the world repeatedly in the time Picasso, right, lived, and his images fractured too. The way he reassembled the shards made the forces that blasted them apart comprehensible. The art was almost incidental. The genius was in the understanding it provided the rest of us

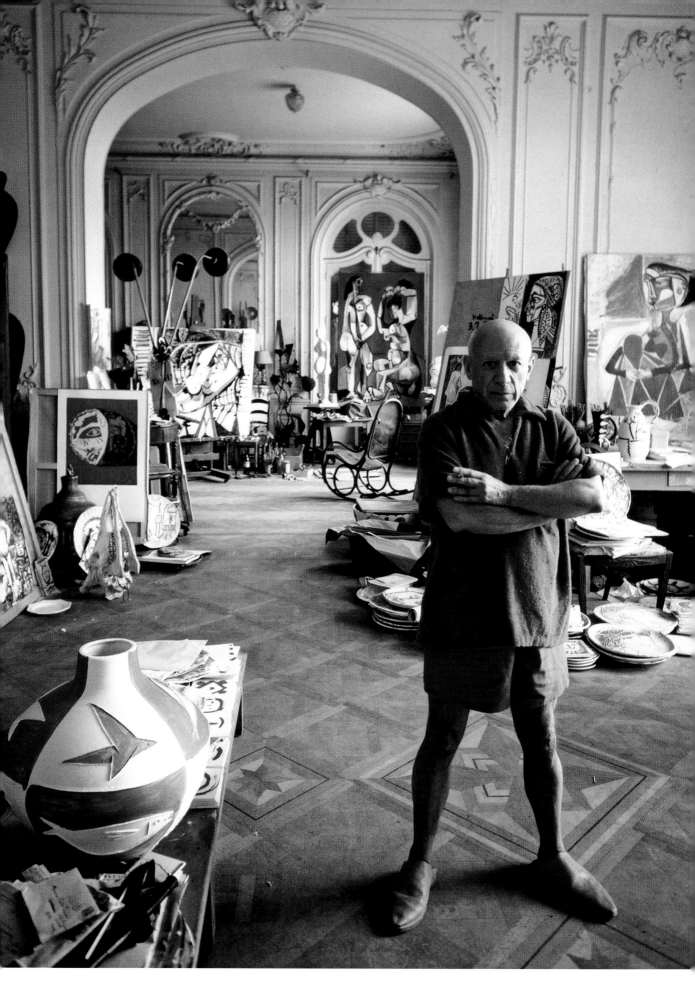

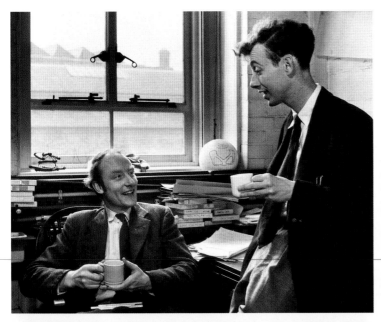

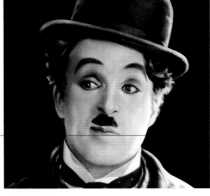

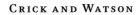

CRICK AND WATSON

One of them (Crick, far left above) had no Ph.D. by age 35. The other (Watson) got his at 19. No matter. In 1953 they strode into the Eagle pub in Cambridge, England, and announced they had discovered what they called the "secret of life." We call it DNA, and it forms the basis of nearly every bit of biological science done today

CHARLIE CHAPLIN

When you're as prolific as he was, you have to start fast. Chaplin, above, made his first short film in 1914—and made 34 more before 1915. Comedy is evanescent; in his long career, he made it permanent. Doubt that? Watch *City Lights* today and try not to laugh throughout it—and not to cry at the end

LOUIS ARMSTRONG

What Satchmo, left, could improvise was better than what a million other jazzmen would spend a life composing. Long after his death, you hear him every time someone else picks up a horn. The cosmos may hear him too: his music was included on a record tucked aboard the Voyager spacecraft

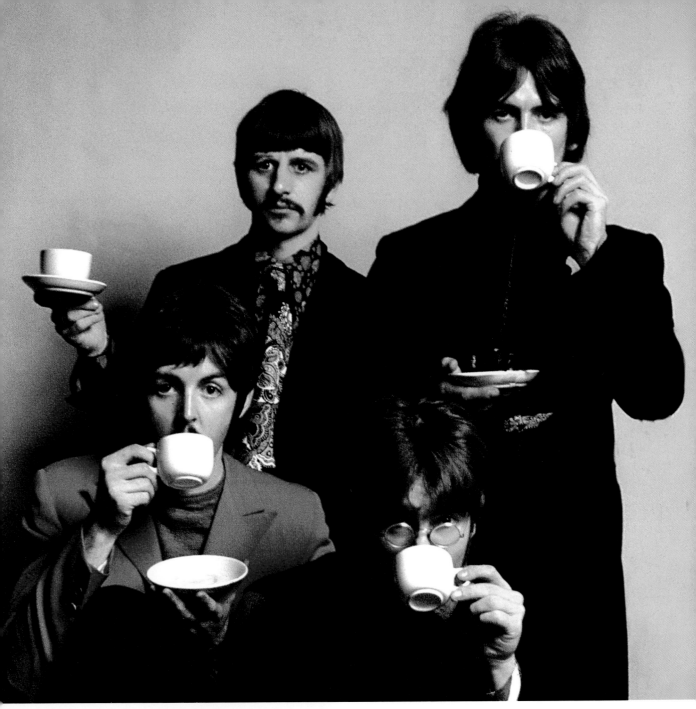

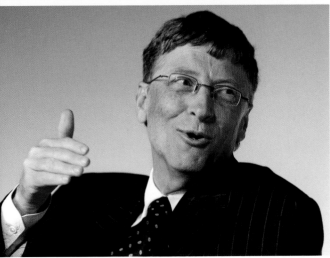

THE BEATLES
The restless talent that made the group what it was later blew it up, as the four musicians went their own ways. But in the time the Beatles, above, were together, it took the genius of the parts to make the incandescence of the whole

BILL GATES
People parsing genius always point to numbers, and Gates, left, has them: the 1590 SAT score, the rumored 170 IQ. But if intelligence is measured by influence, Gates, the father of the PC, may have no modern peer

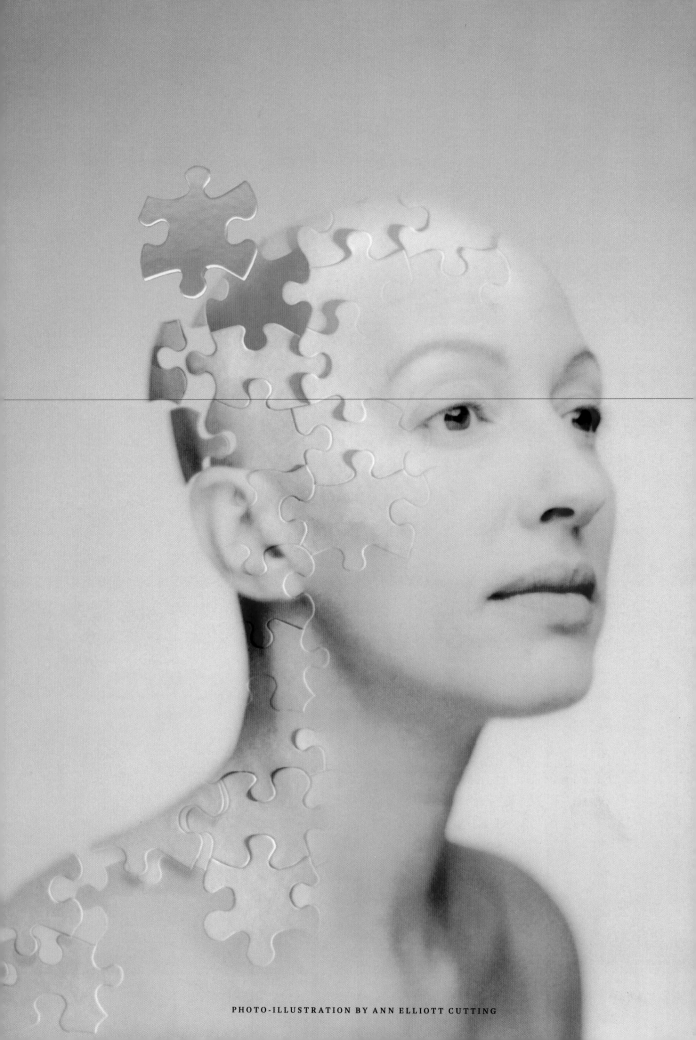

PHOTO-ILLUSTRATION BY ANN ELLIOTT CUTTING

memory

Our ability to recall experiences is one of
our most perishable powers. Why do we
remember so much—and forget so much?

Forgetting Is the New Normal

The more scientists study the workings of memory, the more they understand why it so often fails. The good news: some of what's broken you may be able to fix

BY SUE HALPERN

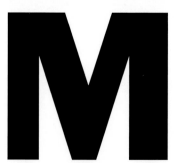

MEMORY RESEARCHER Scott Small would like to reassure you that you're not losing your wits. Visit him in his lab at Columbia University Medical Center, tell him how the last time you went to a party, you couldn't put names to faces, how telephone numbers slip your mind, and he'll walk to his blackboard, pick up a piece of chalk and draw two lines. One, he will tell you, represents age. The other is memory. "As age goes up, memory goes down," he says. "Memory decline occurs in everyone."

Anecdotally, that's no surprise. Approach middle age and it's hard not to notice that your recall is flickering. This, we're reassured, is perfectly normal—all your friends are complaining about the same thing, aren't they?—yet it doesn't feel normal. What's more, while most memory loss is normal, some people become part of the unlucky minority that develops Alzheimer's

Adapted from Can't Remember What I Forgot: The Good News from the Front Lines of Memory Research *by Sue Halpern.* © *2008 by Sue Halpern. Published by Harmony Books, a division of Random House Inc.*

disease or other forms of dementia. Why not you?

Alzheimer's is expected to strike 34 million people globally by 2025 and 14 million in the U.S. over the next 40 years. Half of all people who reach age 85 will exhibit symptoms of the disease. That, however, means the other half won't. And since U.S. life expectancy currently tops out at 80.4 for women and 75.2 for men, by the time your 85th birthday rolls around, you're not likely to be troubled by Alzheimer's disease—or anything else.

Still, that doesn't make it any easier when you forget to pick up the dry cleaning or fumble to recall familiar addresses. Fortunately, science is as interested in what's going on as you are.

Consider for a moment how memory is supposed to operate. Consider, that is, the hippocampus. A cashew-shaped node of tissue, the hippocampus sits deep in the temporal lobe. If the brain has a gatekeeper of sensory information, the hippocampus is it. The aroma of frying bacon, the smooth finish of polished granite, a phone number you need to call—all must pass through the hippocampus. Only if information gets in can it be moved along to the prefrontal cortex, where it will be briefly held in what is called working—or short-term—memory. When you look up the phone number, dial it and promptly forget it, that's your prefrontal cortex working in tandem with your hippocampus.

But let's say you're hanging on to the number 10 min-

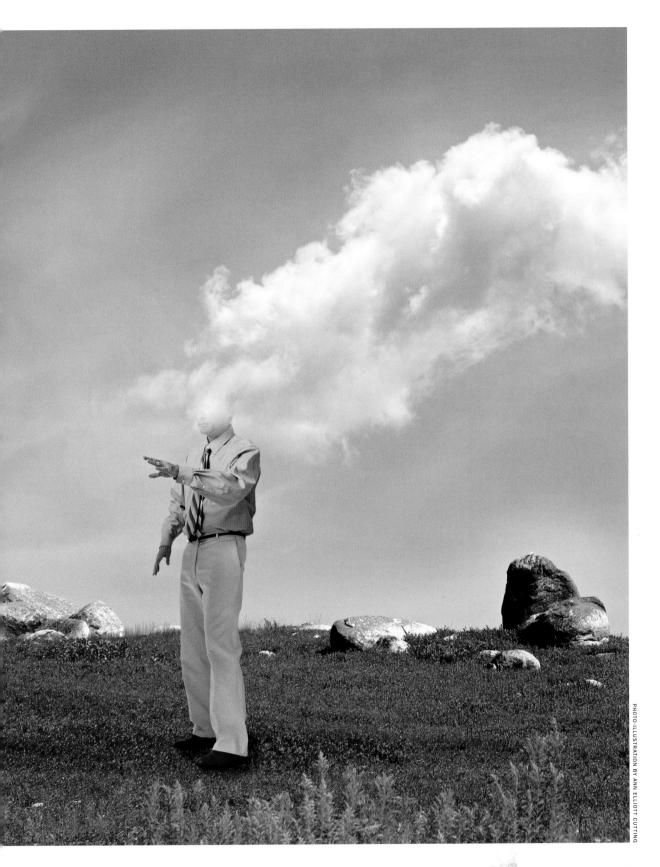

utes or even 10 months later. Why? Because that bit of information has gone through a chemical process called long-term potentiation (LTP) that strengthens the synapses. You need LTP to form long-term memories. And LTP takes place in the hippocampus.

The hippocampus begins to malfunction early in Alzheimer's disease. Imaging studies have shown that people with Alzheimer's typically have a smaller than average hippocampus. As the hippocampus shrinks, the pathway between it and the prefrontal cortex begins to degrade as well. The hippocampus also goes at least somewhat awry in normal memory loss. "It's relatively stable in volume till about 60," Harvard neuroscientist Randy Buckner explains, "and then begins to change. People with Alzheimer's disease, though—they slide off the cliff."

Small and his colleagues have been trying to understand the difference. Small's hunch—now proven—was that a node of the hippocampus different from the one affected in Alzheimer's was breaking down in normal memory loss. "In humans, monkeys and rats," he says, "normal aging targets a node called the dentate gyrus, while a different node—the entorhinal cortex—is relatively spared. But in Alzheimer's disease, it's almost exactly reversed." Small has gone deeper, pinpointing a protein molecule known as RbAp48 that is less abundant in the brains of people suffering ordinary memory loss.

But even if you are low in RbAp48, don't pin all the blame on your hippocampus. As people get older, they have problems paying attention—a function controlled by the prefrontal cortex, which starts to diminish in size well before middle age. It also begins to use the brain's fuel, glucose, less efficiently and loses about half its concentration of the neurotransmitter dopamine.

Amy Arnsten, a neurobiologist at Yale Medical School, has roused idling monkey and rat

Brain Calisthenics

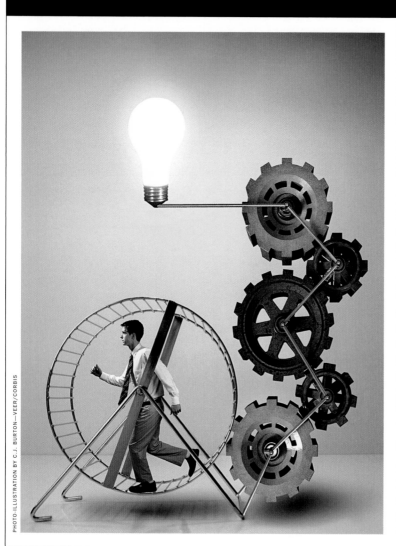

Keeping your brain sharp is similar to keeping your body fit. The mind can be strengthened just like muscles—with regular training and rigorous practice. That doesn't mean spending hours puzzling out complicated brain teasers. Instead, focus on solving a lot of straightforward problems that require short but intense bursts of concentration. Here are a few examples of cognitive drills that can serve as wind sprints for your thinking. If you find your mind feeling sluggish, try repeating similar exercises daily.

QUICK COUNTING

INSTRUCTIONS: Count to 120 out loud in less than a minute. Make sure to articulate the syllables to practice rapid, accurate mind-mouth coordination.

brains with a medication called guanfacine, which appears to amplify the circuits of the prefrontal cortex. The drug has been tested on children with attention-deficit/hyperactivity disorder as well as on people with traumatic brain injury, posttraumatic stress and schizophrenia and in each case has improved memory.

Something else is going on as we get older that also impairs memory: our brains are making fewer neurons. Until a decade ago, the common assumption was that we were born with a fixed number of brain cells that die off as we age, making us, well, dimmer. The brain continues, however, to produce neurons throughout the life cycle, but only in two places: the olfactory bulb and the hippocampus. And not just anywhere in the hippocampus but in the dentate gyrus, the very node that Small has identified as the site of impairment in normal memory loss. So why should memory fade at all? The answer may come from the gym.

A decade ago, when neuroscientist Fred Gage of the Salk Institute made the discovery that the adult brain continues to regenerate, the brains in question belonged to mice. Some of the mice had been sedentary, others had been exercising, and the ones that logged the most miles on their wheels produced many more new neurons.

That appears to be true for humans too. In a 2007 paper, Gage, Small and Columbia University psychologist Richard Sloan revealed that after pounding the treadmill four times a week for an hour for 12 weeks, a group of previously inactive men and women, ages 21 to 45, showed substantial increases in cerebral blood volume (CBV)—a proxy for the growth of new neurons because where there are more cells, there are more blood vessels.

Not only did the CBV profile of the human exercisers mirror that of the mice, but the people who exercised more did better on a slew of memory tests. Other evidence backs this up. In a study of "previously sedentary" older subjects by psychologist Arthur Kramer at the University of Illinois and others at Israel's Bar-Ilan University, investigators found that those who engaged in aerobic exercise did better cognitively than those who stretched and toned but never got their hearts pumping. What's more, subsequent imaging showed that aerobic exercise "increased brain volume in regions associated with age-related decline in both structure and cognition."

Meanwhile, researchers from the Karolinska Institute in Stockholm who have been following over 1,500 people for more than 35 years found a significantly lower rate of dementia, including Alzheimer's, in those who exercise. Another study, of 2,000 elderly men living in Hawaii, showed that those who walked two miles or more a day were half as likely to develop dementia as those who walked a quarter-mile or less.

WORD TRICKS (STROOP TEST)

INSTRUCTIONS: Say the color the word is printed in, not the word itself. Try to say all 10 without a mistake within 15 seconds.

BLUE YELLOW RED GREEN YELLOW
GREEN BLUE RED YELLOW RED

SOUND TRACKING

INSTRUCTIONS: Count the syllables in the phrases below. Can you do it in your head (without using your fingers) in less than 45 seconds?

Reading is to the mind what exercise is to the body. —SIR RICHARD STEELE

Brain: an apparatus with which we think that we think. —AMBROSE BIERCE

Nothing fixes a thing so intensely in the memory as the wish to forget it.
—MICHEL DE MONTAIGNE

RAPID RECALL

INSTRUCTIONS: Memorize these 30 words by studying them for two minutes. Then put away the list and, using a separate sheet of paper, see how many you can remember in two minutes.

circle	pilot	tubing	apple	midnight	sleigh
bread	rope	pottery	mind	bell	folder
dog	office	shape	head	problem	train
sister	map	edge	kite	flap	account
coat	thunder	section	brand	point	wallet

SPEEDY SUMS

INSTRUCTIONS: Complete these 10 simple equations in less than 20 seconds. Seem too easy? Even basic math requires focus.

6×7 $15 - 6$ $13 + 4$ 3×9 $16 \div 4$
$19 - 8$ 8×5 $9 + 6$ $6 \div 2$ 4×8

Sources: *Train Your Brain* by Ryuta Kawashima; *Brain Age* by Nintendo

Memory Quiz

Memory on the fritz? Sometimes it takes a professional to tell you whether you've got a real problem. Below is one test the pros use to measure your recall.

1. Remember these words:
orange telephone lamp

2. Remember this name and address:
Mary Smith, 650 Park Street, Athens, N.Y.

3. Who were the past five U.S. Presidents?

4. Who were the past three mayors of your city?

5. What were the names of the last two movies you saw?

6. What were the names of the last two restaurants in which you ate?

7. Have you had more difficulty than usual recalling events from the previous few weeks?
☐ **Yes** ☐ **No**

8. Have you noticed a decline in your ability to remember lists, such as shopping lists?
☐ **Yes** ☐ **No**

9. Have you noticed a decline in your ability to perform mental math, like calculating change?
☐ **Yes** ☐ **No**

10. Have you been more forgetful about paying bills?
☐ **Yes** ☐ **No**

11. Have you had more trouble remembering people's names?
☐ **Yes** ☐ **No**

12. Have you had more trouble recognizing faces?
☐ **Yes** ☐ **No**

13. Has it become harder to find the right words you want to use?
☐ **Yes** ☐ **No**

14. Have you been having more trouble remembering how to perform simple physical tasks such as operating the microwave or the remote control?
☐ **Yes** ☐ **No**

15. Does your memory interfere with your ability to function:
at work?
☐ **Yes** ☐ **No**
at home?
☐ **Yes** ☐ **No**
in social situations?
☐ **Yes** ☐ **No**

16. Do you recall the three words you were given earlier?

17. Do you recall the name and address you were given?

SCORING: Questions 3-6: one point for each correct answer (12 points). **Questions 7-15:** one point for each "no" answer (11 points). **Questions 16-17:** one point for each correct answer (9 points)

INTERPRETATION: 28-32 points: You have a better-than-average memory. **22-27 points:** You may need follow-up. **0-21 points**: You probably need a professional evaluation

Source: Gayatri Devi, Lenox Hill Hospital

But physical activity isn't all there is to improving your memory. There's also what you eat. Take blueberries. According to Jim Joseph, a neuroscientist with the U.S. Department of Agriculture in Boston, blueberries zap free radicals (highly reactive atoms that can damage tissue), reverse aging, enhance cognition and—this is the kicker—cause new neurons to grow. If you're a rat.

In one animal study, Joseph developed a series of motor-skills tests that he and his associates called the Rat Olympics. Rats had to walk balance beams and stay upright during a log-rolling task. Those that had been raised on blueberry rat chow did better than those that hadn't, leading Joseph to conclude that "blueberries were actually able to reverse motor deficits in these aging animals." More remarkably, when mice that had been genetically altered to express Alzheimer's were put on the blueberry diet, they did not experience memory loss. Joseph's work has shown some similar benefits from walnuts, which contain alpha-linolenic acid, an essential omega-3 fatty acid.

No matter what you eat, if you want to maintain a sharp memory, you should strive for a diet that keeps your belly fat down. A study of more than 6,500 people published in the journal *Neurology* showed that people who were overweight and had a large belly were 2.3 times as likely to develop dementia as those with normal weight and belly size, while those who were obese and had a large belly were 3.6 times as likely. Scientists have long known that as belly fat—which disrupts body chemistry more than less reactive fat elsewhere on the body—increases, blood glucose rises. Some of Small's animal studies show that rising glucose levels in turn disrupt the function of the dentate gyrus. "It's possible," Small says, "that blood glucose is one of the main contributors to age-related memory decline in all of us."

None of these insights, of course, make your sputtering memory less frustrating. And nothing entirely removes the specter of true dementia and the horrors it implies. Still, figuring out how memory works is the most important step in figuring out how it can be fixed. When you can make some of the fixes yourself, the news is even better. ∎

Fretting About Forgetfulness

It's hard not to worry when you notice your memory's slipping. Not all of that anxiety is unwarranted, but much is

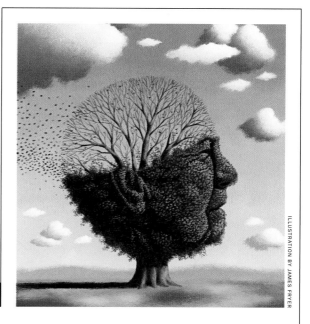

YOU FORGET WHERE YOU PUT YOUR KEYS, often misplace your glasses and certainly can't remember names as well as you used to. At bedtime, you stare haplessly into the bathroom mirror, wondering whether you've already brushed your teeth. Once you showed up for a dinner date at the wrong restaurant. What's happening? Should you regard such lapses as a sign of more serious memory problems, maybe even Alzheimer's?

Not likely. Mental slips like these are a normal part of midlife. Even teenagers, capable of reeling off an entire iPod's worth of lyrics, occasionally blank out. Unless your forgetfulness is accompanied by deeper failures in reasoning and logic, it's nothing to fret about. After all, if being absentminded were a sign of mental disarray, you'd have to write off Einstein, who bungled simple arithmetic even while working on relativity.

You should feel concern if memory loss becomes a consistent pattern—forgetting what you've just said or done, repeatedly missing appointments, telling old jokes again and again or unwittingly making phone calls to the same people about the same subjects. It may also be a sign of trouble if these flubs are followed by changes in behavior, such as irritability, depression or irrational suspicions (your house has been broken into, your spouse is cheating on you).

Even then, don't jump to hasty conclusions. In middle age, many things can cause memory loss or mental fuzziness, to say nothing of confused thinking—menopause, for example. Also keep in mind that age normally takes a toll on what psychologists call processing speed—the rapidity with which you can recall the names of people and places. In some cases, it's a very good thing if some data is periodically erased from memory. Our brains have evolved with a kind of built-in forgetfulness, lest they become hopelessly cluttered with useless information.

In older people, memory problems may also be the result of poor diet, vitamin deficiencies or glandular imbalances (all reversible with treatment) rather than the classic types of dementia associated with age. Even if a physician ultimately diagnoses Alzheimer's disease—which is done by eliminating other possibilities rather than by a direct test, because none is available other than a brain biopsy—the news needn't be as bleak as it once might have seemed.

The mind-robbing disease is still incurable, and the drugs that are currently available only ease certain symptoms like anxiety, confusion and insomnia or slightly slow down its relentless progression. Still, the assault that Alzheimer's launches on the brain varies enormously from person to person. Even five or 10 years after a diagnosis, some people suffer only modest memory loss while retaining old skills like the ability to play golf or sail a boat—or, for that matter, recall long-ago happenings. Alzheimer's, moreover, is one of the hottest areas of scientific research. Scientists are continually identifying genes that appear to be involved in the growth of nerve-cell-killing plaques in the brain. Even if the disease is not curable, it may soon be more treatable than ever. —*By Frederic Golden*

ILLUSTRATION BY JAMES FRYER

77

The Many Flavors of Memories

We recall events in a multisensory way—
and we distort those recollections just as
creatively. Chemistry causes those errors,
but chemistry might fix them too

By Michael D. Lemonick

LIKE JUST ABOUT EVERY ONE OF MY contemporaries, I still remember exactly where I was and what I was doing when John F. Kennedy was shot. It's so vivid, it's almost like watching a movie. I was home sick from fifth grade, lying on the couch in the living room. My mother had a talk-radio station playing. Suddenly a newscaster broke in with the news that shots had been fired in Dallas and the President had been rushed to a hospital. Then a few minutes later came these precise words, spoken in just the tone you would imagine: "Ladies and gentlemen, the President is dead," followed immediately by funereal music. My mother burst into tears, and I, profoundly embarrassed, fled the room.

That scene, which I have replayed in my mind many times since 1963, perfectly illustrates two crucial facts that neurologists have come to understand in the past few years about the workings of human memory. The first is that, despite its movie-like clarity, my memory of J.F.K.'s assassination is almost certainly wrong in some details. That's because I'm not simply calling up the original memory laid down in November 1963. I'm recalling the last time I thought about it. Each time we retrieve and re-store a memory, it can be subtly altered.

What goes back into our brains is like the new version of a text document, overwriting the old.

The second fact: memory and emotion are intimately linked biochemically, with hormones like adrenaline actively involved in both. "Any kind of emotional experience will create a stronger memory than otherwise would be created," says James McGaugh, a neurobiologist at the University of California at Irvine. "We remember our embarrassments, our failures, our fender benders."

On the face of it, that doesn't seem especially surprising: we feel strong emotion at important events, which are obviously more memorable. But the connection is much deeper than that and dates back to our evolutionary past. "The major purpose of memory," observes McGaugh, "is to predict the future." An animal that can remember the significance of that large, nasty-looking thing with the big teeth and sharp claws will survive longer and produce more offspring.

What happens biochemically, says McGaugh, is that when faced with an emotionally charged situation, our bodies release the stress hormones adrenaline and cortisol. Among other things, these signal the amygdala, a tiny, neuron-rich structure nestled inside the brain's medial temporal lobes, which responds by releasing another hormone, norepinephrine. Norepinephrine does two important things. First, it kicks the body's autonomic nervous system into overdrive: the heart beats faster,

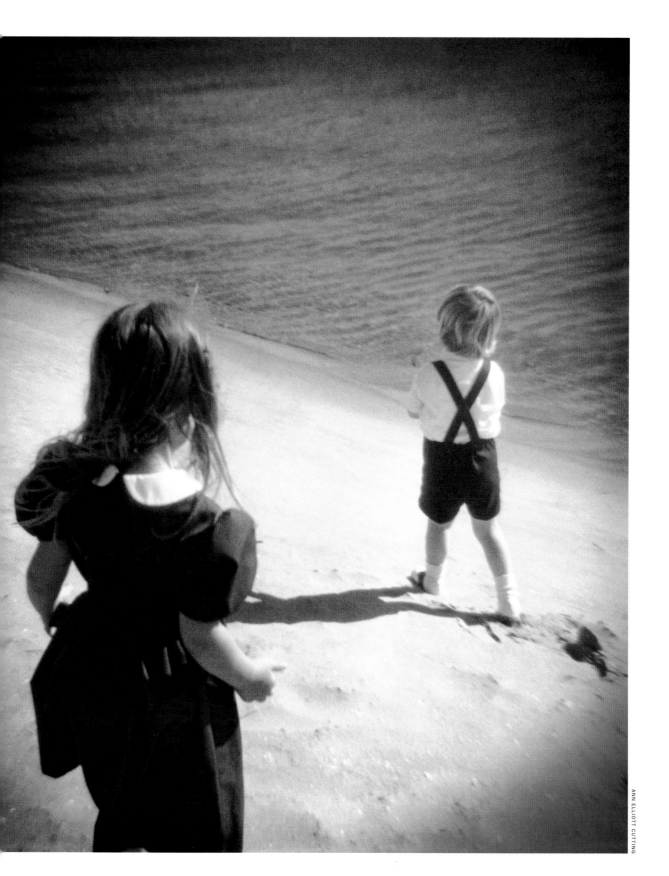

79

respiration quickens, and the muscles tense in anticipation of a burst of physical exertion.

Second, even as it's kick-starting the body, the amygdala sends out a crackle of signals to the rest of the brain. Among other things, these signals tell the neurons that any memories recorded in the next few minutes need to be especially robust. One piece of evidence for this scenario: Lawrence Cahill, a colleague of McGaugh's at Irvine, showed subjects emotionally arousing film clips, simultaneously gauging the activity of their amygdalae using positron-emission tomography (PET) scans. Three weeks later, he gave the subjects a surprise memory quiz. The amount of amygdala activity predicted with unexpected accuracy how well they remembered the film clips.

Imaging studies also make clear that it isn't just dangers or tragic events that cement memory formation. Positive emotions, which are also mediated through the amygdala, have the same effect. Again, that's a perfectly reasonable evolutionary development. If eating or having sex makes you happy, you'll remember that and do it again, keeping yourself healthy and passing on your genes as well.

This is an oversimplification, of course. Other neurotransmitters and even plain glucose—the sugar the brain uses for energy—may also play a part. All of these things work in tandem, which means their complexity multiplies. And then there's the peculiar case of the woman who contacted McGaugh because she remembers absolutely everything. The stress-hormone model does not seem to apply in her case. Says McGaugh: "At some point, I asked if she knew who Bing Crosby was. She's 40, so Bing Crosby doesn't loom large in her life, but she knew he died on a golf course in Spain, and she gave me the date, just like that." Researchers are working to determine if the woman's brain is structurally different from everyone else's.

But aside from such odd cases, virtually no one doubts

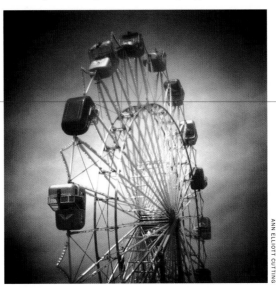

ANN ELLIOTT CUTTING

the connection between emotions and memories—and nobody doubts that memory could be enhanced artificially. That's not likely to work out too well, however. Give someone a shot of adrenaline, and memory may temporarily improve. But the chemical also drives up the heart rate dangerously. Other memory enhancers, like Ritalin or amphetamines, which are used by college students to cram for exams, are highly addictive.

For people who want to modify bad memories, there may be hope. Roger Pitman, a professor of psychiatry at Harvard Medical School, is working to understand post-traumatic stress disorder (PTSD). The syndrome, he believes, is the result of brain chemicals reinforcing themselves in a cerebral vicious circle. "In the aftermath of a traumatic event," he says, "you tend to think more about it, and the more you think about it, the more likely you are to release further stress hormones, and the more likely they are to act to make the memory of that event even stronger."

That's consistent with McGaugh's ideas, but there are only a few bits of evidence so far to support it. One bit comes from Israel, where researchers found that of people who showed up at emergency rooms after traumatic events, those admitted with the fastest heartbeats had the highest risk of later developing PTSD. Additionally, investigators have discovered the surprising fact that after a paralyzing accident, there's a much higher rate of PTSD in people suffering from paraplegia (paralysis of the lower body) than in those who suffer quadriplegia (paralysis of all four limbs), at least partly because quadriplegia severs the link between the brain and the adrenal glands.

To test his theory, Pitman went to the emergency room at Massachusetts General Hospital in Boston and intercepted patients who had suffered serious traumas. He gave some of them propranolol, a drug that interferes with adrenaline uptake. The rest got placebos. He also

Positive emotions cement memories, and that makes sense. If eating and having sex make you happy, you'll remember to do them again, keeping yourself fed and passing on your genes

had them tape-record accounts of the traumas. When he played back the tapes eight months later, eight of 14 placebo patients developed higher heart rates, sweaty palms and other signs of PTSD. None of the patients on propranolol had such responses.

Encouraged by his findings, Pitman undertook a much larger trial of the same technique for erasing memories of traumatic events, but the study stirred some controversy. The President's Council on Bioethics condemned the work as unethical, saying that tinkering with memories risks undermining a person's true identity. Pitman rejects such notions as showing bias against psychiatry. After all, he argues, no one suggests that doctors should withhold morphine from people in acute pain on the grounds that it may erase part of their experience.

Other researchers are looking at PTSD as well. Michael Davis, a professor of psychiatry at Emory University in Atlanta, has studied soldiers returning from Iraq to see whether a drug called D-cycloserine could help prevent PTSD. This compound activates a protein that helps the mind form new, less emotional associations with the original trauma. Studies in rats and humans have shown that it can work—and, says Davis, "psychologists are very excited by it."

That's because the theory behind D-cycloserine's action is consistent with old-fashioned talk therapy and especially with cognitive behavioral therapy (CBT), currently the most effective nondrug technique for dealing with phobias, PTSD and obsessive-compulsive disorder. The idea behind CBT is that the patient examines upsetting ideas and consciously assigns new, more positive associations to them. Even traditional Freudian therapy might achieve something similar, by unearthing old memories and exposing them to the daylight of the doctor's office.

D-cycloserine may simply streamline the talk-driven process. Indeed, says Davis, at least one study showed patients on D-cycloserine getting as much benefit from two sessions as a typical patient would from eight. "That's exactly what they're finding in obsessive-compulsive trials too," he says. There are, moreover, a number of other brain receptors and chemicals that show promise in accelerating the formation of new associations. Says Davis: "What we have now could be the tip of the iceberg."

That's hardly surprising. Even without anything approaching a complete understanding of the human brain, neurologists and psychopharmacologists have come up with dozens of medications to treat schizophrenia, depression and other illnesses. The next batch of psychoactive drugs could provide ammunition against the even more mysterious disorders of memory. ∎

BEEN HERE BEFORE? MAYBE IT'S JUST DEJA VU

It's an eerie experience that just about everyone has had: you walk into a room or find yourself in a conversation, and suddenly you have the overwhelming sense that you've lived this moment already. Psychologists call it *déjà vu*—"already seen," in French—but despite the phenomenon's familiarity, no one had offered a convincing explanation for it.

The mystery may have been solved, thanks to a team of neuroscientists at MIT's Picower Institute for Learning and Memory. Neuroscientists already know memories are actually groups of brain cells linked by strong chemical connections. It's important for the brain to know that some memories are similar to each other, but it's also important to distinguish memories that are similar but not identical. This ability is known as pattern separation.

Researcher Thomas McHugh and senior colleague Susumu Tonegawa engineered a type of mouse that lacked what they believed was the gene responsible for pattern separation and devised an experiment to test the theory. Mice were guided into a box where they would get a mild foot shock; they would react by freezing. Then they were guided into a similar box but not shocked. The altered mice would freeze there too. Normal mice figured things out pretty quickly.

This same circuit and this same gene may explain déjà vu. Every so often, the scientists believe, the pattern-separation system misfires, and a new experience that's similar to an older one seems identical. "It doesn't happen very often to most people," Tonegawa says. But when it does, it's unmistakable. —**M.D.L.**

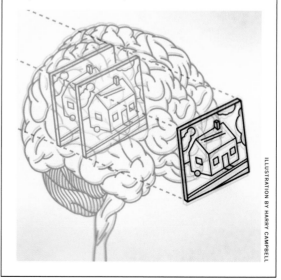

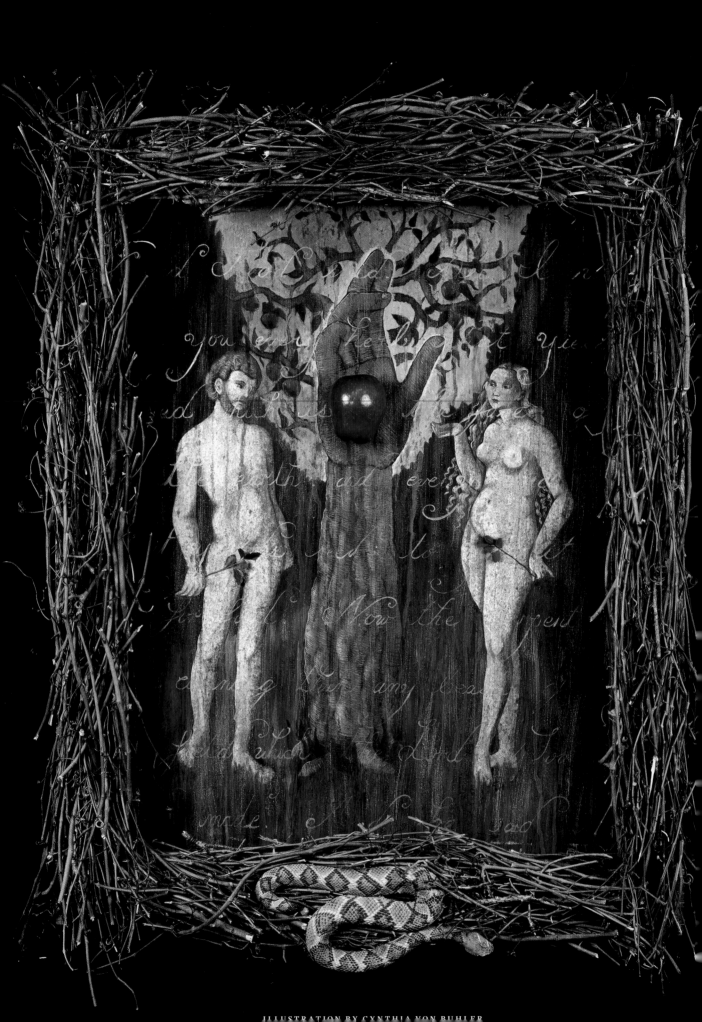

morality

It's hard to fathom how a single species can be so gentle and so wicked. But we're both, and there are deep reasons for our two sides

What Makes Us Moral?

Empathy and goodness are writ as deeply
in our genes as murder and savagery.
We did not choose to have two parts to our
nature, but we can choose which to embrace

By Jeffrey Kluger

F THE ENTIRE HUMAN SPECIES WERE A SINGLE individual, that person would long ago have been declared mad. The insanity would not lie in the anger and darkness of the human mind—though it can be a black and raging place. And it certainly wouldn't lie in the transcendent goodness of that mind—one so sublime, we fold it into a larger "soul." The madness would lie instead in the fact that both of those qualities, the savage and the splendid, can exist in one creature, one person, often in one instant.

We're a species that is capable of almost dumbfounding kindness. We nurse one another, romance one another, weep for one another. Ever since science taught us how, we willingly tear the very organs from our bodies and give them to one another. And at the same time, we slaughter one another. The past 15 years of human history are the temporal equivalent of those subatomic particles that are created in accelerators and vanish in a trillionth of a second, but in that fleeting instant, we've visited untold horrors on ourselves—in Mogadishu, Rwanda, Chechnya, Darfur, Beslan, Baghdad, Pakistan, London, Madrid, Lebanon, Israel, New York City, Oklahoma City—all of the crimes committed by the highest, wisest, most principled species the planet has produced. That we're also the lowest, cruelest, most blood-drenched species is our shame—and our paradox.

The deeper that science drills into the substrata of behavior, the harder it becomes to preserve the vanity that we are unique among Earth's creatures. We're the only species with language, we told ourselves—until gorillas and chimps mastered sign language. We're the only one that uses tools, then—but that's if you don't count otters smashing mollusks with rocks or apes stripping leaves from twigs and using them to fish for termites.

What does, or ought to, separate us, then, is our highly developed sense of morality, a primal understanding of good and bad, of right and wrong. Morality may be a hard concept to grasp, but we acquire it fast. A preschooler will learn that it's not all right to eat in the classroom, because the teacher says it's not. If the rule is lifted and eating is approved, the child will happily comply. But if the same teacher says it's also O.K. to push another student off a chair, the child hesitates. "He'll respond, 'No, the teacher shouldn't say that,'" says psychologist Michael Schulman, co-author of *Bringing Up a Moral Child.* In both cases, somebody taught the child a rule, but the rule against pushing has a stickiness about it, one that resists coming unstuck even if someone in authority countenances it. That's the difference between a matter of morality and one of mere social convention.

The deepest foundation on which morality is built is the phenomenon of empathy, the understanding that what hurts me would feel the same way to you—and we're

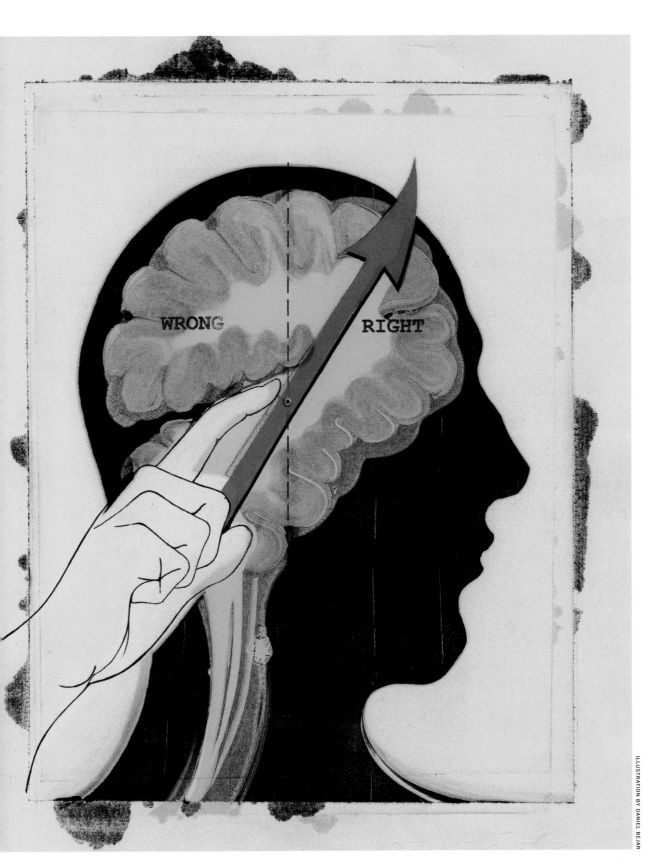

85

not the only species that understands that idea. It's not surprising that animals far less complex than we are would display a trait that's as generous of spirit as empathy, particularly if you decide there's no spirit involved in it at all. Behaviorists often reduce what we call empathy to a mercantile business known as reciprocal altruism. A favor done today—food offered, shelter given—brings a return favor tomorrow. If a colony of animals practices that give-and-take well, the colony thrives.

But even among animals, there's something richer going on. One of the first and most poignant observations of empathy in nonhumans was made by Russian primatologist Nadia Kohts, who studied nonhuman cognition in the first half of the 20th century and raised a young chimpanzee in her home. When the chimp would make his way to the roof of the house, ordinary strategies for bringing him down—calling, scolding, offers of food—would rarely work. But if Kohts sat down and pretended to cry, the chimp would go to her immediately. "He runs around me as if looking for the offender," she wrote. "He tenderly takes my chin in his palm … as if trying to understand what is happening." More recent—less gentle—stories of chimp savagery have muddied the animal's rep for interspecies amity, but a capacity for violence does not preclude a capacity for gentleness too.

Kohts' reports are not the only ones of their kind. Even cynics went soft at the story of Binta Jua, the gorilla who in 1996 rescued a 3-year-old boy who had tumbled into her zoo enclosure, rocking him gently in her arms and carrying him to a door where trainers could enter and collect him.

While it's impossible to directly measure empathy in

O.J. Simpson's 1995 acquittal of double-murder charges may have outraged millions of people, but it did make the morality tale surrounding him far richer, as the culture as a whole turned its back on him

animals, in humans it's another matter. Marc Hauser, professor of psychology at Harvard University and author of *Moral Minds,* cites a study in which spouses or unmarried couples underwent functional magnetic resonance imaging (fMRI) as they were subjected to mild pain. They were always warned before the painful stimulus was administered, and their brains lit up in a characteristic way signaling mild dread. They were then told that they were not going to feel the discomfort but that their partner was. Even when they couldn't see their partner, the subjects' brains lit up precisely as if they were about to experience the pain themselves. "This is very much an 'I feel your pain' experience," says Hauser.

The brain works harder when the threat gets more complicated. A favorite scenario that morality researchers study is the trolley dilemma. You're standing near a track as an out-of-control train hurtles toward five un-

The Virtuous And the Vile

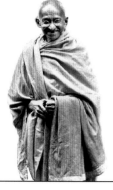

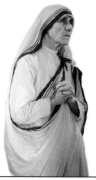

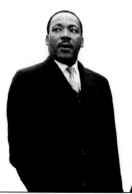

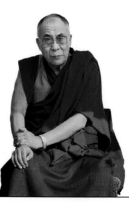

The human pageant is filled with people who have inspired our awe, either for their goodness or their malevolence. The Gandhis and Mother Teresas remind us of our species' potential. Sadly, so do the Pol Pots and Pinochets

MOHANDAS GANDHI
The father of India, he led his country's nationalist movement against British rule with a patient doctrine of nonviolence and peaceful protest

MOTHER TERESA
Born Agnes Gonxha Bojaxhiu, the beatified Roman Catholic nun dedicated her life to educating the disadvantaged and caring for the sick and the poor

MARTIN LUTHER KING JR.
Winner of the Nobel Peace Prize, he led the U.S. out of the shadow of Jim Crow and transformed the country with the power of his vision and words

THE DALAI LAMA
The exiled spiritual leader was also awarded the Nobel Peace Prize, in honor of his nonviolent campaign for Tibetan independence from China

suspecting people—all of whom are related to you, but not members of your immediate family. There's a switch nearby that would let you divert the train onto a siding. Would you do it? Of course. You save five lives at no cost. Suppose your true love is on the siding. Now the mortality score is 5 to 1—but that one is very precious.

Pose these dilemmas to people while they're undergoing fMRI, and the brain scans get messy. Using a switch to divert the train toward an empty track increases activity in the dorsolateral prefrontal cortex—the place where cool, utilitarian choices are made. Complicate things with the idea of diverting the train toward another person, and the medial frontal cortex—an area associated with emotion—lights up. As these two regions do battle, we may make irrational decisions. In a recent survey, 85% of subjects who were asked about the trolley scenarios said they would not kill an innocent person to save five others—even though they knew they had just sent five people to their hypothetical death. In this case, morality trumps the arithmetic of mortality.

How We Stay Good

Merely being equipped with moral programming does not mean we always practice moral behavior. Something still has to boot up that software and configure it properly, and that something is the community. Hauser believes that all of us carry what he calls a sense of moral grammar—the ethical equivalent of the basic grasp of the structure of speech that most linguists believe is with us from birth. But just as syntax is nothing until words are built upon it, so too is a sense of right and wrong useless until someone gives you the tools that allow you to apply it effectively.

It's the people around us who give us those tools. One of the most powerful strategies for enforcing group morals is the practice of shunning. If membership in a tribe is the way you ensure yourself food, family and protection from predators, being blackballed can be a terrifying thing. Religious believers as diverse as Roman Catholics, Mennonites and Jehovah's Witnesses have practiced their own forms of shunning—though the banishments may go by names like excommunication or disfellowshipping.

Sometimes shunning emerges spontaneously when a society of millions recoils at a single member's acts. O.J. Simpson's 1995 acquittal of double-murder charges may have outraged people, but it did make the morality tale surrounding him much richer, as the culture as a whole turned its back on him, denying him work, expelling him from his country club, refusing him service in a restaurant. In 2007, when he attempted to publish a book about the murders, the outcry was so great that not only was the book pulled, the publisher who commissioned the book was fired. She later sued her ex-bosses, alleging that she had been "shunned" and "humiliated." That, the bosses might well have responded, was precisely the point.

"Human beings were small, defenseless and vulnerable to predators," says Barbara J. King, biological anthropologist at the College of William and Mary and author of *Evolving God*. "Avoiding banishment would be important to us."

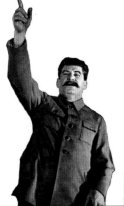 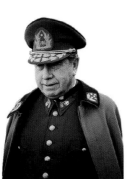 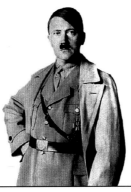 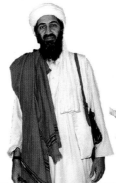 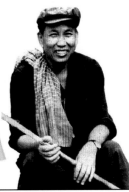

JOSEPH STALIN
As dictator of a vast totalitarian state, the communist chief was responsible for the loss of millions of lives during his quarter-century rule of the Soviet Union

AUGUSTO PINOCHET
After seizing power in a military coup in 1973, the general went on to rule Chile with a murderously iron fist, torturing and killing thousands of his people in the process

ADOLF HITLER
As pure as evil gets, the Nazi dictator launched World War II, engineered the Holocaust and still mystifies scholars studying the capacity for human savagery

OSAMA BIN LADEN
The Saudi millionaire is this century's icon of evil, killing thousands on Sept. 11, 2001, and in earlier attacks on targets that included U.S. embassies and the U.S.S. *Cole*

POL POT
As leader of the brutal Khmer Rouge, he ordered the murders of more than a million people in Cambodia and still insisted, "My conscience is clear." No doubt it was

With so many redundant moral systems to keep us in line, why do we so often fall out of ranks? Sometimes we can't help it, as when we're suffering from clinical insanity and behavior slips the grip of reason. Things are different in the case of someone like a serial killer, a cool and deliberate criminal who knows the meaning of his deeds yet continues to commit them. For neuroscientists, the iciness of the acts calls to mind the case of Phineas Gage, the Vermont railway worker who in 1848 was injured when an explosion caused a tamping iron to be driven through his prefrontal cortex. Improbably, he survived, but he exhibited stark behavioral changes—becoming detached and irreverent, though never criminal. Ever since, scientists have looked for the roots of serial murder in the brain's physical state.

A 2006 study published in the journal *NeuroImage* may have helped provide some answers. Researchers working through the National Institute of Mental Health scanned the brains of 20 healthy volunteers, watching their reactions as they were presented with various legal and illegal scenarios. The brain activity that most closely tracked the hypothetical crimes— rising and falling with the severity of the scenarios— occurred in the amygdala, a deep structure that helps us make the connection between bad acts and punishments. As in the trolley studies, there was also activity in the frontal cortex. The fact that the subjects themselves had no sociopathic tendencies limits the value of the findings. But knowing how the brain functions when things work well is one good way of knowing where to look when things break down.

Fortunately, the overwhelming majority of us never run off the moral rails in remotely as awful a way as serial killers do, but we do come untracked in smaller ways. We face our biggest challenges not when we're called on to behave ourselves within our family, community or workplace but when we have to apply the same moral care to people outside our tribe.

The brutal line we may draw between insiders and outsiders is evident everywhere—mobsters, say, who kill promiscuously yet go on rhapsodically about "family." But it has its most terrible expression in wars, in which the dehumanization of the outsider is essential for wholesale slaughter to occur. Volumes have been written about what goes on in the collective mind of a place like Nazi Germany or the collapsing Yugoslavia. While killers like Adolf Hitler or Slobodan Milosevic can never be put on the couch, it's possible to understand the xenophobic strings they play in their people.

"Yugoslavia is the great modern example of manipulating tribal sentiments to create mass murder," says Jonathan Haidt, associate professor of psychology at the University of Virginia. "You saw it in Rwanda and Nazi Germany too. In most cases of genocide, you have a moral entrepreneur who exploits tribalism for evil purposes."

That, of course, does not take the stain of responsibility off the people who follow those leaders—a case that war-crimes prosecutors famously argued at the Nuremberg trials and a point courageous people have made throughout history as they sheltered Jews during World War II or refuse to murder their Sunni or Shi'a neighbor.

For grossly imperfect creatures like us, morality may be the steepest of all developmental mountains. Our opposable thumbs and big brains gave us the tools to dominate the planet, but wisdom comes more slowly than physical hardware. We surely have a lot of killing and savagery ahead of us before we fully civilize ourselves. The hope—a realistic one, perhaps—is that the struggles still to come are fewer than those left behind. ∎

Where Decisions Are Made

Understanding the intricacies of our most complicated organ is a scientific work in progress, but there is some consensus on how the brain tackles moral dilemmas. These are some of the major regions involved in moral decision-making

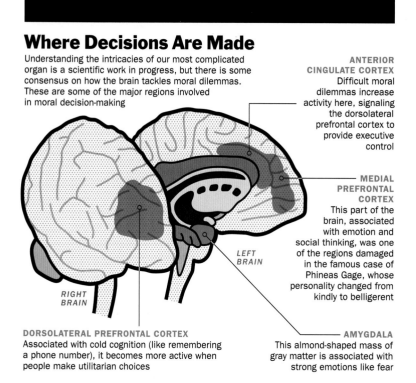

ANTERIOR CINGULATE CORTEX
Difficult moral dilemmas increase activity here, signaling the dorsolateral prefrontal cortex to provide executive control

MEDIAL PREFRONTAL CORTEX
This part of the brain, associated with emotion and social thinking, was one of the regions damaged in the famous case of Phineas Gage, whose personality changed from kindly to belligerent

LEFT BRAIN

RIGHT BRAIN

DORSOLATERAL PREFRONTAL CORTEX
Associated with cold cognition (like remembering a phone number), it becomes more active when people make utilitarian choices

AMYGDALA
This almond-shaped mass of gray matter is associated with strong emotions like fear

Moral Dilemmas

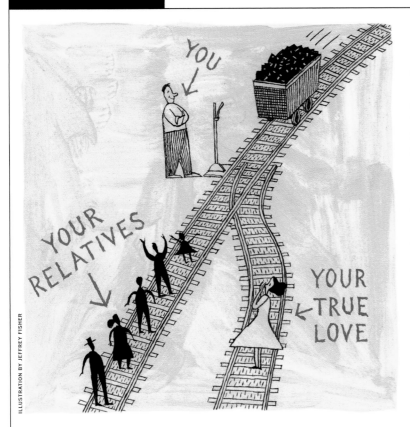

The Runaway Trolley

A runaway trolley is headed down a track toward five of your relatives—none of whom are immediate family members. They can't be warned in time to get out of the way. You are standing near a switch that would divert the trolley onto a siding, but your true love is standing there and also can't be warned in time. Could you throw the switch, killing one precious person to save five less precious ones? Suppose you were standing on an overpass and could save the five people only by pushing your love down onto the tracks? (Assume that jumping onto the tracks yourself is not an option.)

DIVERT TRAIN	YES	NO
PUSH LOVER	YES	NO

The Crying Baby

It's wartime, and you're hiding in a basement with your baby and a large group of other people. Enemy soldiers are patrolling outside and will be drawn to any sound. Your baby starts to cry loudly and cannot be stopped. Smothering him to death is the only way to silence him and save the lives of everyone else in the room. Could you do so? Assume instead that the baby is not yours, that the parents are dead or unknown and that there will be no criminal penalty for killing him. Under those changed circumstances, could you be the one who smothers the baby if no one else would?

YOUR BABY	YES	NO
SOMEONE ELSE'S BABY	YES	NO

The Sinking Lifeboat

You are adrift in a life raft after your cruise ship has sunk. There are too many survivors for all the rafts, and yours is dangerously overloaded. You are certain to sink, and even with life vests on, all the passengers are sure to die because of the frigid temperature of the water. One person on the boat is awake and alert but gravely ill and certain not to survive the journey no matter what. Throwing that person overboard would lighten the raft enough to prevent it from sinking and save the lives of everyone else on board. Could you be the one who tosses the person out?

I COULD THROW A SURVIVOR OVERBOARD	YES	NO

The Kidney Transplant

You have two children, both of whom will die tomorrow without a kidney transplant. You are the only possible donor—but assume you can donate only one kidney. You have a crystal ball and can see that Child A will grow up to be a successful surgeon and will save many lives herself. She is so sick now, however, there is only a 50% chance she will survive the transplant. Child B will grow up to be a gambler, and while she will never hurt anyone, she will never help anyone either. There is a nearly 100% chance she will survive the transplant and live a healthy life. To whom would you give your kidney?

CHILD	A	B

Race and The Raging Brain

Nothing justifies the scourge of racism, but human history at least explains it. We're wired to like people who are like us. How does that turn into hating everyone else?

BY JEFFREY KLUGER

N 2009, AN AFRICAN-AMERICAN PRESIDENT held a Passover seder in the White House. Chew on that for a second. Time was, such a scene was not just improbable; it was laughable—literally—the kind of setup a Borscht Belt comedian or late-night TV host would use for an easy punch line. And laughter was the best you could have hoped for. Let too many people think too long about the real prospect of a black President's hosting a Jewish ceremony in the U.S. Executive Mansion and, well, it doesn't pay to contemplate the kinds of demons you might unleash.

But that was then, this is now, and President Barack Obama's historic seder registered as a one-day, three-paragraph story tucked somewhere inside the morning newspaper. The fact that the moment made so little news might be bigger news than the seder itself.

The human species is not always a rational one, but we have managed to move along in a ragged march that for all its setbacks has been a steady climb from savagery to civilization, from subsistence to the grand achievements of art and science and philosophy. And in the midst of all that, there's been the bloody matter of race.

Like many other animals, we are a species that comes in a whole palette of colors. Unlike all other animals, however, we have a complex brain that allows us to assign complex meanings to those colors. White skin is good, brown skin is worse, and black skin is worst of all—unless, of course, you're black or brown, in which case things run the other way.

It's not color alone that drives us apart. When we're not tribalizing ourselves by race, we're doing so by religion, by language, by history, by geography. So Hutu slaughter Tutsi, Nazis massacre Jews, Turks kill Armenians, and Catholics and Protestants, Sunnis and Shi'ites, Christians and Druze fight back-and-forth wars that last for generations and resolve nothing at all. But it's race that historically divides us most starkly. What is it about color that inflames and divides us so? Why is it that so inconsequential a thing can summon such demons from such deep places? Answers do exist—in our history, in our families, in our genes, in our brains. And more and more, researchers are teasing them out.

Whatever else you can say about humanity's racist ways, the fact is, we come by them naturally. There are few species on the planet that aren't aware of the concept of friend and foe, us and other. "You see it all the way down to tadpoles, which preferentially associate with other tadpoles depending on how closely related they are," says biologist Jay Phelan of UCLA, a co-author of the book *Mean Genes*. "Animals are good at this, they're fast at it, and it's pretty clear what the adaptive value is."

Humans are no different, nor would we want to be. The moment you get old enough to toddle away from the

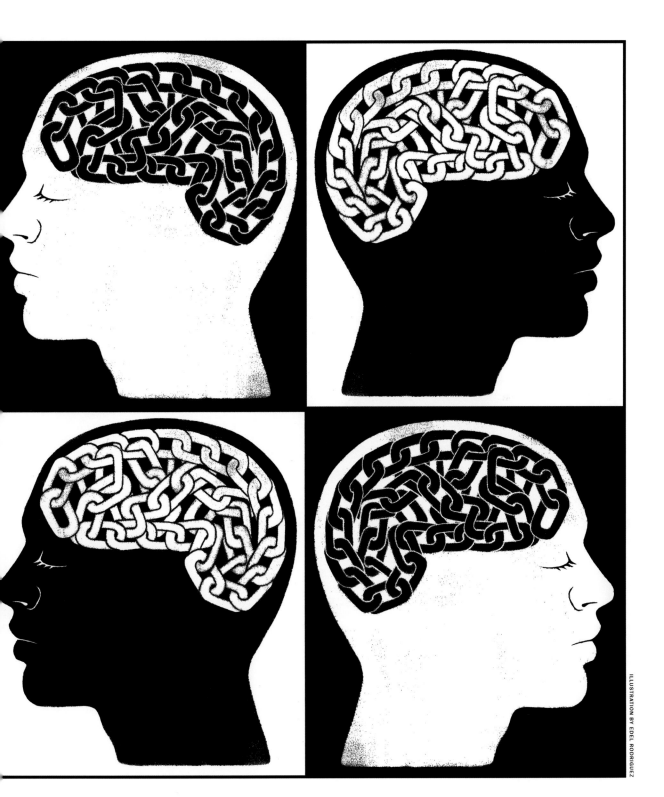

91

communal campfire, you'd better be able to distinguish between the individuals you know—and who mean you no harm—and the ones you don't. "Historically, we lived in small bands but would sometimes come into contact with people in other bands," says anthropologist Yolanda Moses of the University of California at Riverside. "The whole idea of us and them is part of being *Homo sapiens*."

The problem with such an otherwise adaptive tendency is that once we draw those lines, we can't help falling in love with us and growing cool to them. It's not enough for your home group to be the one you know best; it also must actually be the best. The language of your tribe is more lyrical than the gibberish other tribes speak; your music is sweeter than that noise you hear coming from across the valley. Similarly, your men are stronger, your women lovelier, your clothes prettier, your food tastier.

"You want some psychological mechanism to make your group cohesive," says developmental psychologist Yarrow Dunham of the University of California at Merced. "The features that define groups vary a lot, but once they are defined, you prefer your own. And when someone belongs to your group, you like that person better too."

So inclined are humans to divide themselves into clans that even when groups don't naturally exist, we invent them. We identify ourselves by our clubs, our communities, our political parties. Army duels Navy for supremacy in football. The Crips kill the Bloods for supremacy in

the streets. Baseball lovers in Boston describe themselves not as just fans but as nothing short of a Red Sox nation. "There is something very basic about in-group and out-group distinctions," says social psychologist John Bargh of Yale University. "Groups succeed or fail together."

Sometimes, affiliations can be created by something as inconsequential as an article of clothing. Dunham recently conducted a study in which he divided preschoolers into two groups according to the color of T shirt he gave them to wear, then read them stories about each group. Later on, the kids were much likelier to remember the good things that had been said about their own group and the less good things said about the other. "Kids show these preferences right away, in the lab, on the spot," Dunham says.

Preschoolers, of course, can always change the color of their T shirt, but it's a lot harder to change the color of your skin. Before the 1500s, most humans were unable to travel far enough from their homeland to encounter people of other races. When we did, our brains went slightly nuts. The human mind is what research psychologist Joshua Correll of the University of Chicago calls a "meaning-making machine." Constantly pelted by information, it needs to make order of the storm, and one of the best ways to do that is by sorting things. There are big things and small things, loud things and soft things, hot things and cold things. "The categories may

Changing the Mind-Set on Race

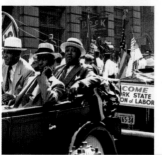

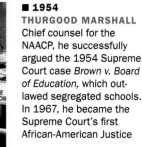

■ 1954
THURGOOD MARSHALL
Chief counsel for the NAACP, he successfully argued the 1954 Supreme Court case *Brown v. Board of Education,* which outlawed segregated schools. In 1967, he became the Supreme Court's first African-American Justice

■ 1939
MARIAN ANDERSON
The great contralto was barred from performing at a concert hall because of her race. With the aid of the White House, she got a bigger venue: the Lincoln Memorial, where she delivered a history-making Easter performance

■ 1941
A. PHILIP RANDOLPH
A grandfather of the civil rights movement, Randolph was a labor organizer, best known for unionizing railroad porters— a traditionally black position. It was at a quiet meeting in 1941, however, that he changed history, proposing the first march on Washington, which finally occurred in 1963

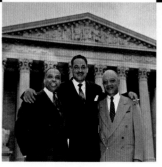

■ 1955
ROSA PARKS
Fed up with riding at the back of the bus because of her race, she took a seat at the front. She was arrested, but the 382-day bus boycott that followed led to the abolition of the discriminatory law and demonstrated the power of organized protest

not all be real," says Moses, "but they're a way of trying to understand things."

One of the most powerful categories we use is color—sensible in a world in which we must learn such basic ideas as blood is red, and that means danger; the sky is blue, and that means up; and Mom was wearing her yellow sweater, which can help you spot her if you get lost at the mall. "When children enter preschool, color is one of the first things they learn," says Jessica Henderson Daniel, a Harvard University psychologist who was part of a team that recently completed a study of racial self-awareness among young African Americans. "We tell children that it's a sign of being smart."

Once you start seeing colors, it's hard to stop. In 2008 investigators at the Max Planck Institute in Munich conducted a revealing study in which they showed one group of volunteers pictures of objects such as carrots and bananas in their proper color and showed another group the same pictures in an ambiguously muddy shade. When they were asked about the pictures later, both groups recalled seeing the objects in the correct color, even though only one of the groups had. In other words, if you learn a carrot is orange, you'll always see a carrot as orange; color trumps truth in a way that wholly exaggerates its meaning. Now imagine the shock when black people, white people, red people and brown people—all of them hardwired to overvalue color this

way—began venturing out and meeting one another.

In the U.S. these meetings were especially fraught. The encounters didn't happen over time, with a slow commingling of browner people bumping into whiter people and both groups retreating to their home camps until they could make sense of it all. Rather, white Europeans came to North America en masse and there encountered an existing population of red people. Not long after, European Americans began importing enslaved Africans, adding another skin tone to the continental color wheel. "They were all plopped down right next to each other, and they saw the differences between them as bigger than they were," says Jeffrey Long, a human geneticist at the University of Michigan who specializes in global DNA diversity.

Making things worse was the disparity in power, with industrialized Europeans possessing weapons and tools lacked by people adapted to agrarian lives. This made it easy for whites to dismiss Native Americans as savages, poor stewards of their land who deserved to have it taken from them. Africans, similarly, were brutes by nature and might actually benefit from the discipline slavery provided. Handily, whites were also willing to change the justifications as circumstances warranted. After emancipation, says psychologist John Dovidio of Yale, blacks were described no longer as brutish but as childlike and simple, justifying the Jim Crow laws

■ **1961**
FREEDOM RIDERS
Black and white protesters boarded interstate buses to visit the South and test compliance with the 1960 *Boynton v. Virginia* decision, which outlawed segregation in bus terminals. Violence and arrests greeted their arrival, particularly in Birmingham, Ala., where the riders were attacked

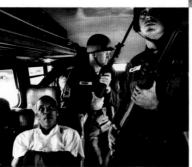

■ **1963**
MARTIN LUTHER KING JR.
The goal of a march on Washington was achieved in 1963 and was a signal moment in American history. A quarter-million people attended, and millions more watched on TV as King delivered his "I Have a Dream" speech

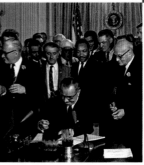

■ **1964**
LYNDON B. JOHNSON
His presidency ended badly, but it began brilliantly, as Johnson signed the Civil Rights Act banning segregation in schools, jobs and housing. In 1965, he followed with the Voting Rights Act, ensuring that blacks were not denied the power of the ballot

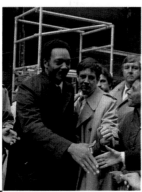

■ **1984**
JESSE JACKSON
Before Barack Obama, there was Jackson. He ran for President in 1984 and 1988, and while he failed to win the Democratic nomination, he collected more than 13 million votes. The idea of an African-American President would never seem so alien again

that followed. "Stereotypes," says Dovidio, "respond to a function they're serving."

Worse, they tend to stick around. In 1998 psychologist and social scientist Mahzarin Banaji of Harvard co-created what's known as the Implicit Association Test (IAT), a tool for exploring the instant connections the brain draws between races and traits. Previously administered only in the lab but now available online (implicit. harvard.edu), the IAT asks people to pair up pictures of white or black faces with positive words like *joy, love, peace* and *happy* or negative ones like *agony, evil, hurt* and *failure.* Speed is everything, since the survey tests automatic associations. When respondents are told to link the desirable traits to whites and the undesirable ones to blacks, their fingers fairly fly on the keys. When the task is switched, with whites being labeled failures and blacks labeled glorious, fingers slow considerably, a sure sign the brain is struggling.

When Banaji, along with cognitive neuroscientist Liz Phelps of New York University, conducted brain scans of subjects using functional magnetic resonance imaging, they discovered one of the reasons for the results. White subjects shown images of black faces responded with greater activation of the amygdala—a region deep in the brain that processes such feelings as alarm and fear—than when they were shown white faces. Later studies showed similar results when black subjects looked at white faces.

Happily, the brain is not all amygdala, and there are higher regions that can talk sense to the lower ones. Phelps cites studies showing that when blacks and whites were flashed pictures of opposite-race faces only subliminally—blinked at them so quickly that the subjects weren't consciously aware of seeing them—the amygdala reacted predictably. When the images were flashed more slowly so that the subjects could process them consciously, the amygdala still lit up, but so did the anterior cingulate and the dorsolateral prefrontal cortex, regions that calm automatic responses.

But what about when the brain goes the other way? What about when racism explodes into full-blown hatred—with all the violence that can go with it?

81%

Percentage of U.S. population (excluding Native Americans) that was white in 1790. Whites now represent 68% and will fall below the majority by 2050

12%

Percentage of U.S. population that is black, down from 19% in 1790. An additional 2% is mixed race

15%

Percentage of U.S. population that is Latino— the largest nonwhite group. For census purposes, not a race but an ancestral group

Any species capable of what anthropologists call cold hate may be a species beyond help. **But scientists are hopeful that we can change, especially as they learn that race, as people understand it, doesn't even exist**

History's monsters—the Hitlers, Karadzics, Pol Pots, Stalins—may kill on a scale far vaster than do small-bore thugs like Klansmen or church bombers, but they all kill, usually with relish. It's hard to know how ordinary human brains become so decoupled from empathy, but the problem almost certainly begins with the very complexity of those brains.

Brains of other animals operate mostly in the present and past. When they encounter an outsider, like a member of an opposing group, simply driving off the interloper is sufficient, since they don't give much thought to whether the intrusion will happen again. Humans think of time in a more three-dimensional way, operating with a sense of the future and the ability to plan for it. That spells trouble for perceived enemies, with one group setting out to eradicate a threat by using the straightforward method of eradicating the other group. And as our ability to develop weapons has progressed, our ability to carry out those murderous plans has too. "For the same aggressive impulse, we can do a lot more killing," Dovidio says.

But why do some societies—or individuals—cross the line into savagery and others don't? Psychologist Robert Sternberg, dean of the College of Arts and Sciences at Tufts University, believes three things are necessary.

First comes what psychologists call a negation of intimacy—a snuffing out not only of empathy for members of the target group but also of the belief that they even deserve empathy since they may not be wholly human. It's no coincidence that the Hutu in Rwanda referred to the Tutsi as cockroaches and Nazi propaganda films depicted Jews as rats. Even good people will burn a hornet's nest.

The second component is what Sternberg labels *passion,* which is—more than mere contempt for the hated group—a deep, visceral loathing. "Passion is hot hate," he says, "the kind you see in road rage."

Finally, there's commitment, a cognitive, intellectual-

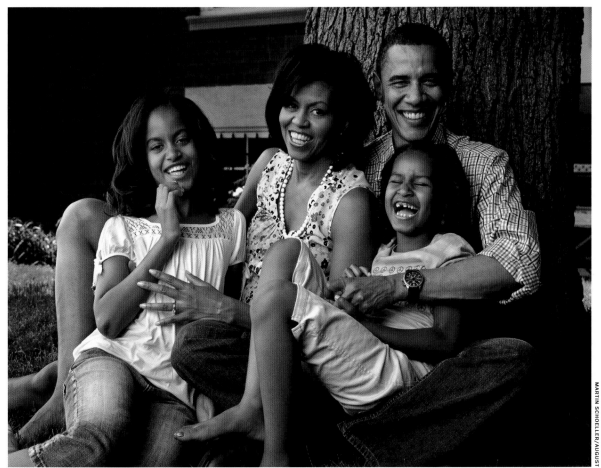

National symbols *Cultures have many ways of showing themselves to the world. In the 21st century, this is the face of the American family*

ized decision to act, often justified by the belief that the target group is guilty of some grievous historical wrong, like winning the other group's land in a long-ago war. "Commitment," says Sternberg, "is more of a cold hate."

Any species capable of a thing called cold hate might be a species beyond help, but scientists are hopeful we can change. One way might be to begin to embrace what anthropologists already know, which is that race, at least as we think we understand it, doesn't even exist. The physical traits that seem to distinguish races so profoundly are based on only a tiny handful of unremarkable genetic sequences that tell you little of any value about the people carrying them.

Judging by current U.S. trends, people may be accepting this newer view of things intuitively, if not scientifically. In 2003, Phelan co-authored an admittedly controversial study in which he measured the ankles, fingers, feet, ears and wrists of biracial students and found them to be more symmetrical than those of monoracial students. What's more, other subjects, shown pictures of mixed-race and single-race people, consistently found the mixed-race pictures more attractive. In a culture that prizes prettiness, Phelan believes this is one small sign that the walls dividing us are collapsing.

Even now, that collapse may be accelerating. The global giddiness that greeted the election of Obama was certainly not shared by everyone. Tens of millions of people voted against him—most for political and policy reasons, some certainly for racial ones. But every single one of the people whose vote was based on race has now been bathed in images of an African-American man as the most powerful person in the world, his African-American wife as head of the nation's First Family, and their African-American daughters as symbols of the country's children. The brain habituates to anything over time. And the next black presidential candidate will not be nearly as much of a jolt.

It is surely too much to hope for a truly color-blind species—or for a single election to erase the meaning of race in even a single country. But it's not too much to hope that humanity's long, ragged march is slowly taking us in that direction. ■

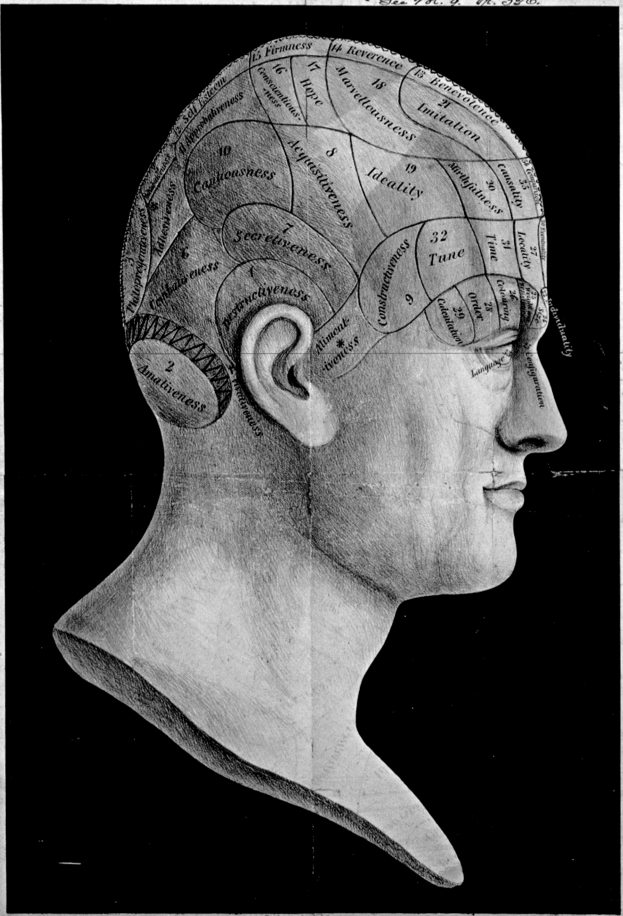

DR. SPURZHEIM.

Divisions of the Organs of Phrenology marked externally.

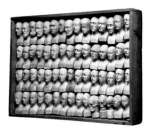

THE WORLD WITHIN

It often seems that we've been trying to understand our brains for as long as we've had them. An organ capable of art and insight, of wisdom and wonder, ought to look the part—somehow spangly and luminous. Instead, it's gray and lumpish. No wonder our efforts to fathom its workings have so frequently gone awry

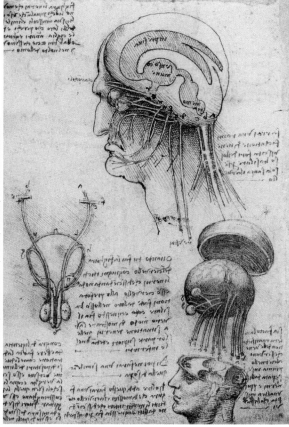

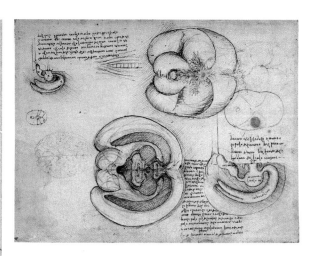

CONTOURS OF THE CRANIUM

Popular in the 1800s, the faux science of phrenology claimed that the brain was divided into regions that governed skills and that the skull conformed to the brain's shape. Bumps on the skull revealed areas in which people excelled. Brain maps, far left, and skull models, top, helped phrenologists interpret heads

MEDIEVAL MASTERPIECES

Leonardo da Vinci was among the first to explore the structure of the brain in real detail. By the late 1400s, he was already developing an understanding of the brain's ventricles, or channels, above, as well as its nerves, left. In a free hour, perhaps, he also diagrammed the male urological system

97

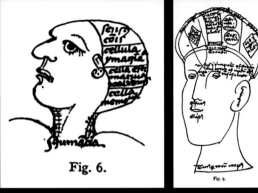

Fig. 6.

Fig. 9.

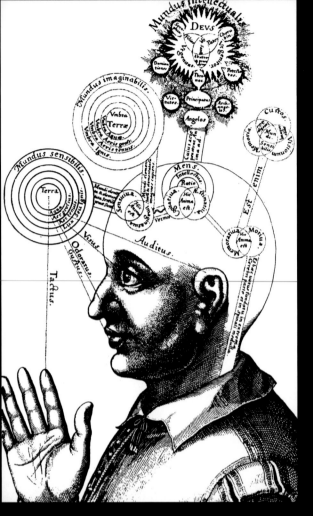

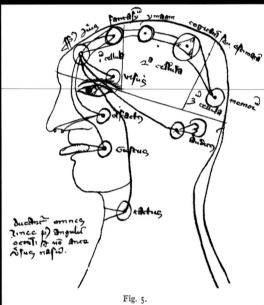

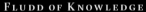

Fig. 5.

FLUDD OF KNOWLEDGE

Robert Fludd was a physician in 16th and 17th century England. His brain maps, above, were based on his belief that the brain reflected the workings of the universe. In the 1400s, anatomists took a more reductionist view, top center and right, dividing the brain into regions that controlled memory, fantasy and more

RESERVOIRS OF EXPERIENCE

Thoughts feel fluid, so they must somehow flow. A 1347 drawing, above right, was an attempt to map the mind's currents. A more detailed effort was made by Carthusian monk Gregor Reisch in 1504, right. Reisch and others believed thoughts flowed in order through three chambers: sensory, reasoning and memory

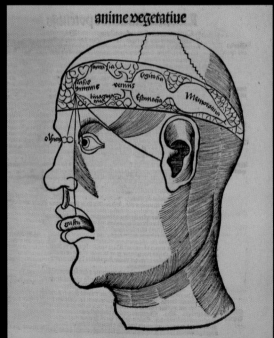

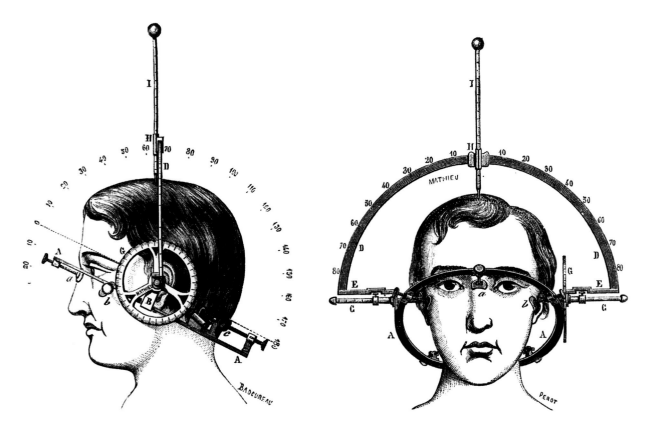

SIZE MATTERED—TOO MUCH

The cephalometer, above—used for measuring the head—was shown in an 1883 text. Today such devices can help guide delicate brain surgery; in the past, skull size was used as a measure of intelligence or to assert racial superiority

TORTURED MINDS

The tranquilizing chair, below left, was an 18th century device thought to soothe mental patients. Exorcism, below, in an 11th or 12th century relief, was an attempt to drive out possessing forces

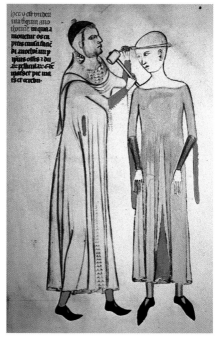

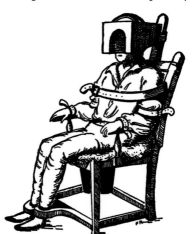

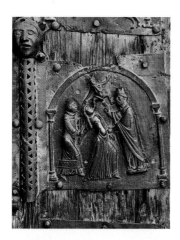

STRAIGHT TO THE SOURCE

One of science's worst ideas, trepanning, above, involved drilling or scraping away the skull to treat mental disorders, migraines, seizures and more. The illustration here is from 1345, but the practice dates back 12,000 years. The criblike object at right does not have the excuse of being nearly so ancient. Designed to control mental patients, it was used in New York in the late 19th century

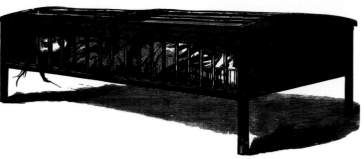

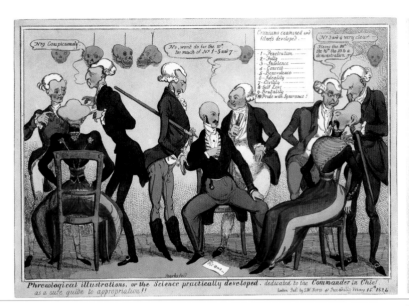

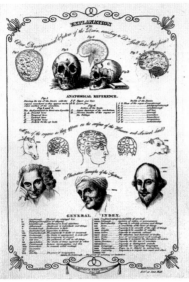

MENTAL MAPMAKERS

The effort to survey the brain's various regions pressed on in 19th century England. Above left, elegant phrenologists examine the skulls of two military men and discuss their findings. The chart above divides mental faculties into various skills, such as math, imagination and wit—the last of these illustrated by Shakespeare

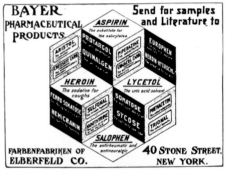

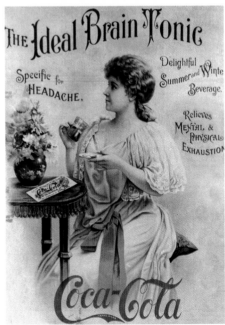

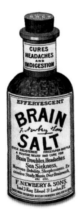

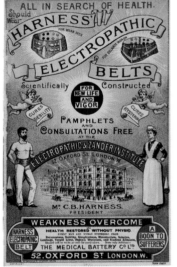

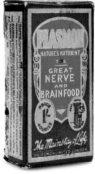

PHARMACOLOGICAL FREE-FOR-ALL

Feeling run-down? How about some heroin? That's just one of the nostrums on offer in an 1890s Bayer ad, top far left. Coca-Cola was advertised as a brain tonic, left, and no wonder: at one time, its makers weren't kidding about the coca part. Brain salt, above left, was said to treat "nervous debility." Plasmon, above right, was a "great nerve and brain food." The electropathic harness, above center, was said to work for lumbago and weak backs, which makes some sense, as well as for hysteria and nervousness, which doesn't

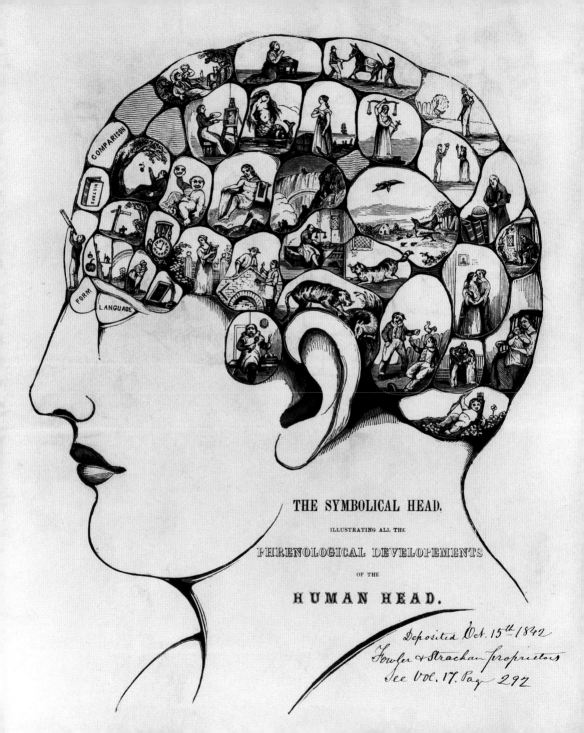

THE SYMBOLICAL HEAD,

ILLUSTRATING ALL THE

PHRENOLOGICAL DEVELOPEMENTS

OF THE

HUMAN HEAD.

Deposited Oct. 15th 1842
Fowler & Strachan Proprietors
See Vol. 17. Page 292

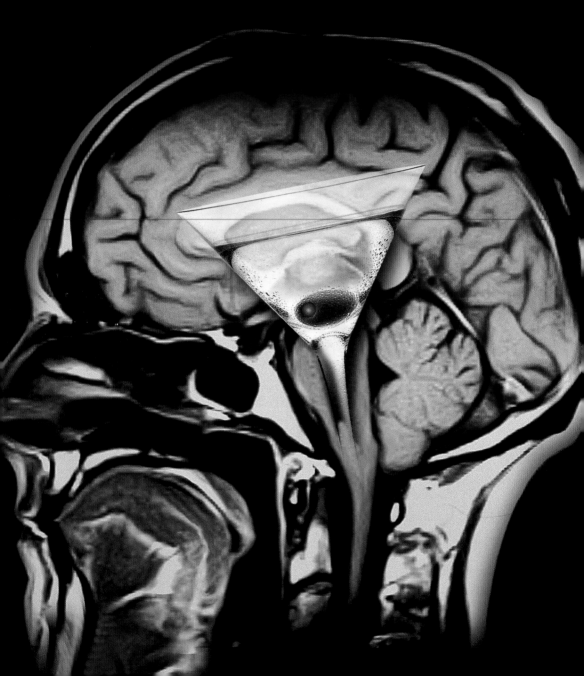

addiction

The world is full of pleasures, and the human brain is wired
to enjoy them all. Sometimes, though, that wiring takes over

When Your Brain Can't Say No

It would be nice if addiction were really just a matter of poor willpower. It's not. It's about neurochemistry gone badly awry—often with deadly consequences

By Michael D. Lemonick

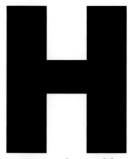

ERE'S A TROUBLING TRUTH about getting drunk: It's fun. Here's a troubling truth about doing drugs: It's fun too. The same holds for eating too much or gambling too much or having too much sex. And here's a more troubling truth about all of them: They can wreck your life—and sometimes end it.

Human beings like to feel good, and like all organisms, we find it hard to stop doing the things that make us feel that way—even after they start making us feel very, very bad. That, at its most basic, is addiction. As long ago as 1950, the American Medical Association declared that alcoholism—perhaps our best-understood addiction—was not a moral failing but a disease. Its physical basis was a complete mystery. Treatment consisted mostly of talk therapy, maybe some vitamins and usually a strong recommendation to join Alcoholics Anonymous (AA). Although it's a totally nonprofessional organization, founded in 1935 by an ex-drunk and an active drinker, AA has managed to get millions of people off the bottle, using group support and a program of accumulated folk wisdom.

While AA is astonishingly effective for some people, it doesn't work for everyone; studies suggest it succeeds about 20% of the time, and other forms of treatment, including various types of behavioral therapy, do no better. The rate is much the same with drug addiction, which experts see as the same disorder triggered by a different chemical. "The sad part is that if you look at where addiction treatment was 10 years ago, it hasn't gotten much better," says Dr. Martin Paulus, a professor of psychiatry at the University of California at San Diego. "You have a better chance to do well after many types of cancer than you have of recovering from methamphetamine dependence."

That could all be about to change. During those same 10 years, researchers have made extraordinary progress in understanding the physical basis of addiction. They know now, for example, that the 20% success rate can shoot up to 40% if treatment is ongoing (very much the AA model, which is most effective when members continue to attend meetings long after their last drink). Armed with an array of increasingly sophisticated technology, including functional MRIs and PET scans, investigators have begun to figure out exactly what goes wrong in the brain of an addict—which neurotransmitting chemicals are out of balance, and what regions of the brain are affected. They are developing a more detailed understanding of how deeply and completely addiction can hijack the brain, by hijacking memory-making processes and by exploiting emotions. Using that knowledge, they've

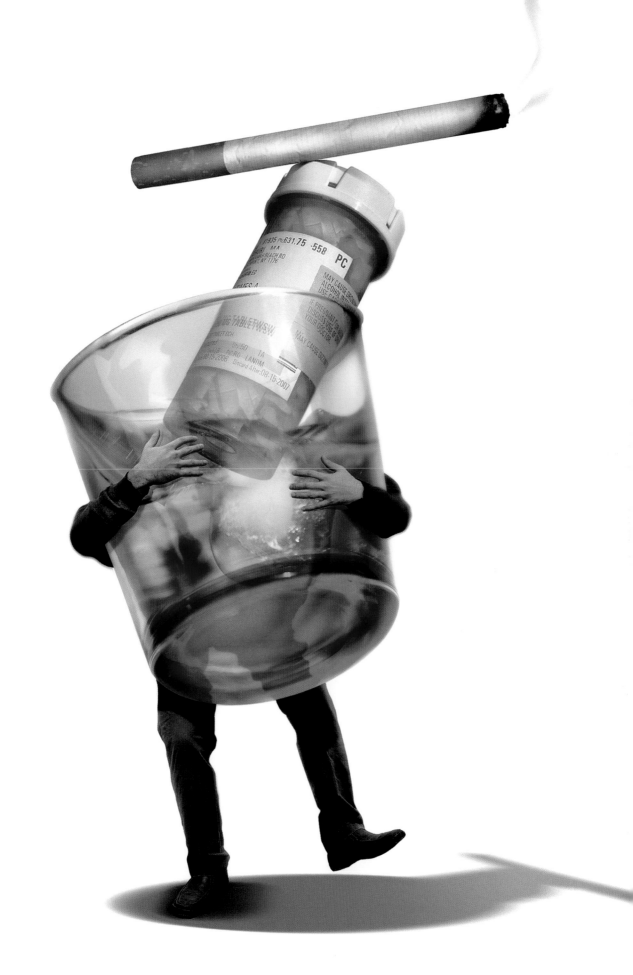

Glucose metabolism

←Lower activity   Higher activity→

Frontal
lobes

Normal subject

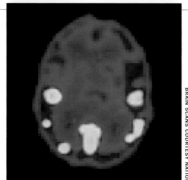

Cocaine abuser 10 days after abuse stops

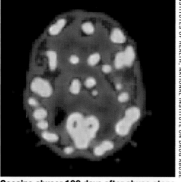

Cocaine abuser 100 days after abuse stops

A peek inside an addict's head
The brain is a chemical machine, and drugs are a monkey wrench. Cocaine reduces glucose metabolism, which is the brain's energy system. The worst effect is in the frontal lobes, where planning, abstract thinking and the regulation of impulses are governed. Quitting the drug can reverse the damage

BRAIN SCANS COURTESY NATIONAL INSTITUTES OF HEALTH, NATIONAL INSTITUTE ON DRUG ABUSE

if it's hard to drive safely under the influence, imagine trying to run from a saber-toothed tiger or catch a squirrel for lunch. And yet, says Dr. Nora Volkow, director of NIDA and a pioneer in the use of brain imaging to understand addiction, "the use of drugs has been recorded since the beginning of civilization."

That's because drugs of abuse co-opt the very brain functions that allowed our distant ancestors to survive in a hostile world. Our minds are programmed to pay extra attention to what neurologists call salience—that is, special relevance. Threats, for example, are highly salient, which is why we instinctively try to get away from them. But so are food and sex because they help the individual and the species survive. Drugs of abuse capitalize on this ready-made programming. When exposed to drugs, our memory systems, reward circuits, decision-making skills and conditioning kick in—salience in overdrive. "Some people have a genetic predisposition to addiction," says Volkow. "But because it involves these basic brain functions, everyone will become an addict if sufficiently exposed to drugs or alcohol."

That can go for nonchemical addictions as well. Behaviors, from gambling to shopping to sex, may start out as habits but slide into addictions. Sometimes there might be a behavior-specific root to the problem. Volkow's research group has shown, for instance, that pathologically obese people who are compulsive eaters exhibit hyperactivity in the areas of the brain that process food stimuli. For them, activating these regions is like opening the floodgates to the pleasure center.

Of course, not everyone becomes an addict. That's because we have other, more analytical regions that can evaluate consequences and override mere pleasure-seeking. Brain-imaging is showing exactly how that happens. Paulus, for example, looked at methamphetamine addicts enrolled in a VA hospital's intensive four-week rehabilitation program. Those who were more

begun to design new drugs that are showing promise in cutting off the craving that drives an addict irresistibly toward relapse—the greatest risk facing even the most dedicated abstainer.

"Addictions," says Joseph Frascella, director of the division of clinical neuroscience at the National Institute on Drug Abuse (NIDA), "are repetitive behaviors in the face of negative consequences, the desire to continue something you know is bad for you."

Addiction is such a harmful behavior that evolution should have long ago weeded it out of the population:

likely to relapse in the first year after completing the program were also less able to complete tasks involving cognitive skills and less able to adjust to new rules quickly. This suggested that those patients might also be less adept at using analytical areas of the brain while performing decision-making tasks. Sure enough, brain scans showed that there were reduced levels of activation in the prefrontal cortex, where rational thought can override impulsive behavior. To his surprise, Paulus found that 80% to 90% of the time, he could accurately predict who would relapse within a year simply by examining the scans.

Another area of focus for researchers involves the brain's reward system, powered largely by the neurotransmitter dopamine. One particular group of dopamine receptors, called D3, seems to multiply in the presence of cocaine, methamphetamine or nicotine, making it possible for more of the drug to enter and activate nerve cells. "Receptor density is thought to be an amplifier," says Frank Vocci, director of pharmacotherapies at NIDA. "[Chemically] blocking D3 interrupts an awful lot of the drugs' effects."

But just as there are two ways to stop a speeding car—by easing off the gas or hitting the brake pedal—there are two different possibilities for muting addiction. If dopamine receptors are the gas, the brain's own inhibitory systems act as the brakes. In addicts, this natural damping circuit, called gamma-aminobutyric acid (GABA), appears to be faulty. Without a proper chemical check on excitatory messages set off by drugs, the brain never appreciates that it's been satiated.

As it turns out, vigabatrin, an antiepilepsy treatment that is marketed in 60 countries (but not yet in the U.S.), is an effective GABA booster. In epileptics, vigabatrin suppresses overactivated motor neurons that cause muscles to contract and go into spasm. Could GABA in the brains of addicts help them control their drug cravings? So far, in animals, vigabatrin prevents the breakdown of GABA so that more of the inhibitory compound can be stored in whole form in nerve cells. That way, more of it can be released when those cells are activated by a hit of a drug.

Hormones may play a role in how people become addicted as well. Studies have shown, for instance, that women may be more vulnerable to cravings for nicotine during the latter part of the menstrual cycle, when the egg emerges from the follicle and the hormones progesterone and estrogen are released. "The reward systems of the brain have different sensitivities at different points

SOME OF THE WAYS WE GET OURSELVES HOOKED

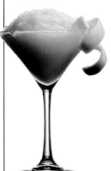

ALCOHOL About 18.7 million people in the U.S. are dependent on or abuse alcohol. Every day, 12,000 more Americans try their first drink.

DRUGS An estimated 3.6 million Americans are drug-dependent, and every day, 8,000 try drugs for the first time. More than half of those first-time users are female and under 18. Marijuana, cocaine and pain relievers are the leading drugs of abuse.

TOBACCO A little bit of good news here, with fewer than 20% of Americans now smoking and the numbers falling. Still, in a population of 300 million, that means tens of millions are hooked on a product that—used as intended—will certainly sicken them and quite possibly kill them.

GAMBLING Winning produces a high, losing means a low, and about 2 million Americans are hooked on that cycle. An additional 4 million to 8 million of us are problem gamblers.

FOOD We need it to survive, but 4 million Americans eat compulsively and addictively—including about 15% of mildly obese people.

SHOPPING One in 20 Americans is hooked on it; stereotypes aside, both genders are equally affected. Advertising exacerbates the problem.

CAFFEINE The most widely used mind-altering drug in the world—and an entirely legal one. Up to 90% of Americans consume it every day, primarily in coffee or soda. Between 40% and 70% of those who try to quit experience withdrawal symptoms.

SEX Compulsive sexual behavior affects 16 million Americans. A third of them are women, and 60% of all sex addicts were abused during childhood.

INTERNET There is disagreement over whether this can be a true addiction, though it can disrupt relationships as severely as compulsive gambling can.

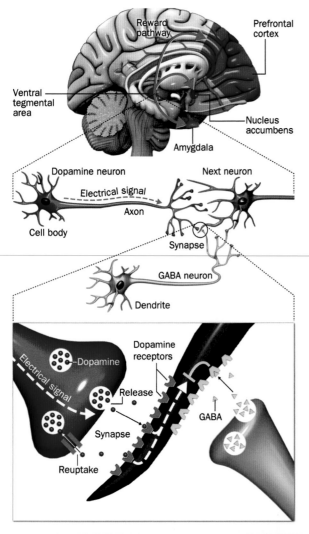

What Happens in the Brain

1. We feel good when neurons in the rewards pathway release a neurotransmitter called dopamine into the nucleus accumbens and other brain areas.

2. The neurons that lie along that reward route communicate by sending electrical signals down their axons. The signal is passed on to the next neuron across a gap called a synapse.

3. Dopamine's job in this process is to ferry the signal across the synapse. When it reaches the opposite side, it binds to receptors in the receiving neuron, producing a jolt of pleasure. Excess dopamine is taken back up by the sending neuron. Other nerve cells release GABA, an inhibitory neurotransmitter that prevents the receiving neuron from becoming overstimulated.

4. Addictive drugs prevent the reabsorption of excess dopamine and block the production of GABA. The result: a high. But addiction can follow, as the normal production of neurotransmitters becomes badly disrupted and the drug is needed merely to keep the user from experiencing the pain of withdrawal.

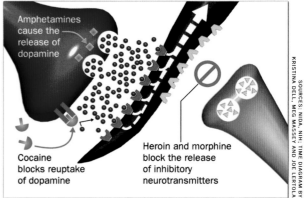

in the cycle," notes Volkow. "There is way-greater craving during the later phase."

That led researchers to wonder about other biological differences in the way men and women become addicted and, significantly, respond to treatments. For years, researchers had documented the way female alcoholics tend to progress more rapidly to alcoholism than men do. This telescoping effect, they now know, has a lot to do with the way women metabolize alcohol. Females are endowed with less alcohol dehydrogenase—the first enzyme in the stomach lining that starts to break down the ethanol in liquor—and less total body water than men are. Together with estrogen, these factors have a net concentrating effect on the alcohol in the blood, giving women a more intense hit with each drink.

But it's the brain, not the gut, that continues to get most of the attention, and one of the biggest reasons is technology. It was in 1985 that Volkow first began using PET scans to record trademark characteristics in the brains and nerve cells of chronic drug abusers. After the subjects had been abstinent for a year, Volkow rescanned their brains and found that they had begun to return to their predrug state. Good news, certainly, but only as far as it goes.

"The changes induced by addiction do not just involve one system," says Volkow. "There are some areas in which the changes persist even after two years." One area of delayed rebound involves learning. Somehow, in methamphetamine abusers, the ability to learn some new things remained affected after 14 months of abstinence. "Does treatment push the brain back to normal," asks NIDA's Frascella, "or does it push it back in different ways?"

One thing science is increasingly validating is the power of the 90-day rehabilitation model, which was stumbled upon by AA (new members are advised to attend a meeting a day for the first 90 days) and is the duration of a typical stint in a drug-treatment program. It turns out that this is just about how long it takes for the brain to reset itself and shake off the immediate influence of a drug. Researchers at Yale University have documented what they call the sleeper effect—a gradual re-engaging of proper decision-making and analytical functions in the brain's prefrontal cortex—after an addict has abstained for at least 90 days.

This work has led to research on cognitive enhancers, or compounds that may amplify connections in the prefrontal cortex to speed up the natural reversal. Such enhancement would give the higher regions of the brain a fighting chance against the amygdala, a more basal region that plays a role in priming the dopamine-reward system when certain cues suggest imminent pleasure—anything from the sight of white powder that looks like cocaine to spending time with friends you used to drink with. It's that learned association that unleashes a craving.

What we learn we can unlearn in other ways too, and scientists studying addictions are increasingly picking up cues from scientists studying an entirely different condition: phobias. It turns out that phobias and drugs exploit the same struggle between high and low circuits in the brain. People placed in a virtual-reality glass elevator and treated with the antibiotic D-cycloserine were better able to overcome their fear of heights than those without benefit of the drug. Says Vocci: "I never thought we would have drugs that affect cognition in such a specific way."

Such surprises have even allowed experts to speculate about whether addiction can ever be cured. That notion goes firmly against current beliefs. A rehabilitated addict is always in recovery because *cured* suggests that resuming drinking or smoking or shooting up is a safe possibility—whose downside could be devastating. But there are hints that a cure might not in principle be impossible. A recent study showed that tobacco smokers who suffered a stroke that damaged the insula (a region of the brain involved in emotional, gut-instinct perceptions) no longer felt a desire for nicotine.

That's exciting, but because the insula is so critical to other brain functions—perceiving danger, anticipating threats—damaging this area isn't something you would ever want to do intentionally. With so many of the brain's systems entangled with one another, it could prove impossible to adjust only one without throwing the others into imbalance.

Even in the age of brain scans and neurotransmitter research, the best way not to drink—or smoke or do drugs—is, well, just not to do it. That's not the high-tech answer, but it is—for now at least—the best answer. ■

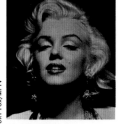

Marilyn Monroe

Addicts in Art and Life The drama of addiction
has long been fodder for filmmakers—partly because so many actors have been addicts themselves. Marilyn Monroe lost her life to an overdose. W.C. Fields, famous for his taste for alcohol, did not begin drinking until his 30s, though he made up for lost time. The stories of struggle and loss unfold in the tabloids and on the screen.

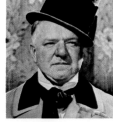

W.C. Fields

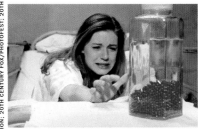

Valley of the Dolls, 1967 *Patty Duke in a pop hit about actresses hooked on pills*

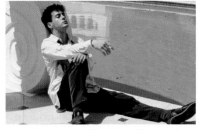

Less Than Zero, 1987 *Robert Downey Jr. battled addiction onscreen and in real life*

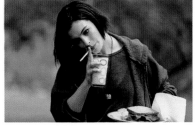

Rachel Getting Married, 2008, *Anne Hathaway starred: an addict, a wedding, a mess*

Science And Your Appetite

You order dessert when you know you shouldn't; you eat French fries instead of a salad. Habits like these aren't good for your diet, but they helped the species survive

By Jeffrey Kluger

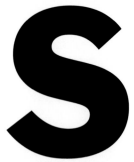

OMEWHERE IN YOUR BRAIN, there's a cupcake circuit. How it works is not entirely clear, and you couldn't see it even if you knew where to look. But it's there all the same—and it's a very powerful thing. You didn't pop out of the womb prewired for cupcakes, of course, but long ago, early in your childhood, you got your first taste of one, and instantly a series of sensory, metabolic and neurochemical fireworks went off.

The mesolimbic region in the center of your brain—the area that processes pleasure—lit up. The vagus nerve flashed signals to the stomach, which began to secrete digestive acids. The pancreas began churning out insulin. As all those complex processes were unfolding, your midbrain filed away a simple, primal, unconscious idea: Cupcakes are good.

Human beings have always had a complicated relationship with food. Staying alive from day to day requires our bodies to keep a lot of systems running just so, but most of them—circulatory, respiratory, neurological, endocrine—operate automatically. Eating is different. Like sex, it's a voluntary thing. And like sex, it's a sine qua non to keep the species going. So nature cleverly rigs the game, making sure we pursue both by making sure we can't resist them.

If you're among the 200 million Americans who have ballooned past their target weight, you can take some consolation from the fact that your early ancestors would be very proud of you. "We were hardwired to eat and eat—and particularly to eat fatty foods because we didn't get them often," says Sharman Apt Russell, author of *Hunger: An Unnatural History*.

Certainly, the body works hard to keep itself balanced. Over the course of a year, the average adult male consumes about 900,000 calories, yet his weight may not rise or fall by more than a pound. Since a pound equals about 4,000 calories, that means his annual intake is just 0.4%—or 11 calories a day—above or below precisely what he needs to keep going. "You are within a potato chip a day of matching your intake with expenditure," says Randy Seeley, professor of psychiatry and associate director of the Obesity Research Center at the University of Cincinnati. It takes a lot to maintain such a precisely balanced cycle of fueling and burning, and what's behind much of it is a substance called ghrelin.

Identified in 1999, ghrelin is produced in the gut in response to meal schedules—and, according to some theories, the mere sight or smell of food—and is designed to give rise to the empty feeling we recognize as a need to eat. When ghrelin hits the brain, it heads straight for

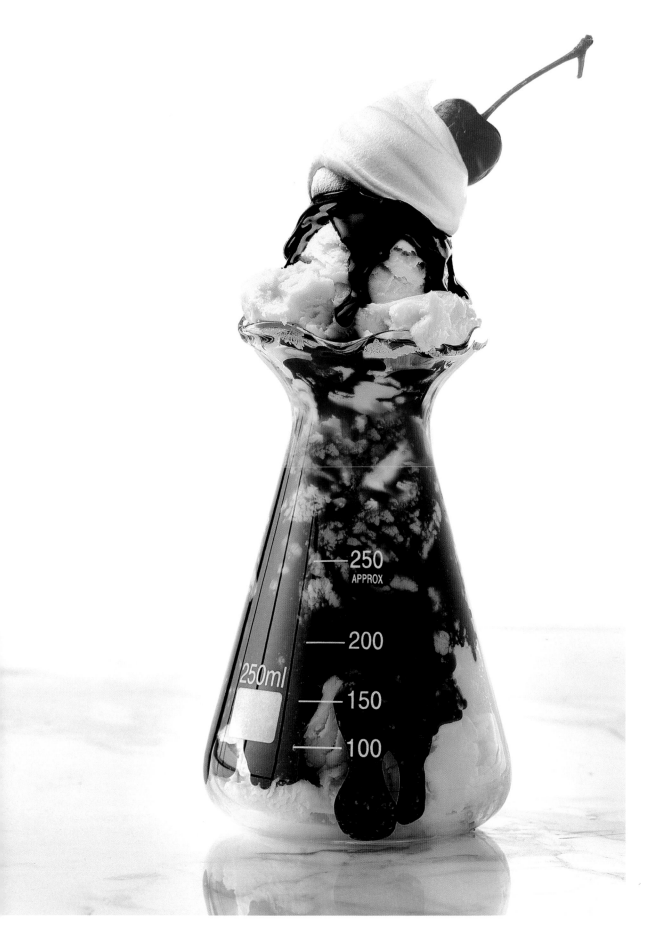

three areas: the hindbrain, which controls the body's automatic, unconscious processes; the hypothalamus, which governs metabolism; and the mesolimbic reward center in the midbrain, where feelings of pleasure and satisfaction are processed.

If ghrelin were all there was to it, we would eat ourselves to death. But even as one system is gunning our hunger higher, another is standing by to slow things down. The first step in that appetite-taming process occurs in the stomach and upper intestine, where nerves that sense stretching and distension alert the brain that you're getting full. That message is reinforced by one peptide and two hormones that first tell your brain you've had enough and then tell your stomach to stop moving food into the intestines—where the real business of digestion takes place—until what's there already has been broken down some. Those are all complex chemical processes, but the message we consciously receive is a much simpler one: Stop eating and push away from the table.

If, despite all those obstacles in the path of overeating, you still pack in too much food—and as a result pack on too much fat—the body has one other, much bigger gun it can roll out: leptin. An appetite-suppressing hormone discovered in 1994, leptin enters the bloodstream and travels to the hypothalamus—one of the brain regions targeted by ghrelin. There it seeks out a pair of neuropeptides known to stimulate appetite and partly muffles their signals.

So with all these metabolic speed bumps in place, why do we ever overeat—never mind compulsively overeat? Michael Cowley, a neuroscientist and an associate professor of physiology and pharmacology at the Oregon National Primate Research Center, is studying how excessive eating mirrors the patterns of drug addiction. Here too, ghrelin appears to play a role. While the hormone affects three areas of the brain, it hits the mesolimbic reward region particularly powerfully. Studies of this part of obese people's brains reveal a level of activity remarkably similar to that in the brains of drug addicts when they are exposed to their preferred substance.

For people struggling with obesity and other consequences of too much food and too much brain chemistry encouraging them to eat it, solutions to the problem are much more important than causes. Diet and exercise are the usual suggestions, and they can work. But the same scientists who have discovered the power of leptin, ghrelin, peptides and hormones to dial our appetite up and down are also looking for ways to harness that power so we can take better control of it on our own. Just as when our ancestors were learning to eat on the savanna, our health and even survival may be at stake. ∎

67%

Portion of U.S. population that is overweight or obese. That includes 17% of children ages 6 to 19

5 BILLION

The total number of pounds by which the 300 million people of the U.S. are currently overweight

17 lb.

The amount by which the average American is overweight. The extra pounds are not, of course, evenly distributed, and many people carry far more

The Decision

1. PANGS

Role Hunger isn't just in your head. When your stomach is empty, it contracts, sending signals along the vagus nerve to the brain

Effect Hunger affects both voluntary and involuntary physical systems. You can ignore the contractions, but a host of other signals will soon take over

2. SENSES

Role The smell and sight of food can stimulate appetite. Your body also wants a variety of sensations, which is one reason you want dessert after a steak

Effect Closing your eyes or walking away may help, but only temporarily. Your body knows when you typically eat and you'll get hungry at those times each day

LOOKS GOOD

3. GHRELIN

Role This hormone, produced in the stomach, sends strong feelings of hunger to the brain. It's rising ghrelin concentrations that account for hunger as mealtimes approach

Effect The more ghrelin, the more hunger you feel. Gastric-bypass surgery reduces ghrelin production, helping obese patients feel full longer

EAT!

4. STRETCHING

Role As you eat, your stomach and intestines begin to stretch, sending nerve impulses to the brain that quiet appetite

Effect It's a slow process. Your stomach may say stop eating, but your brain won't hear the message for several more minutes

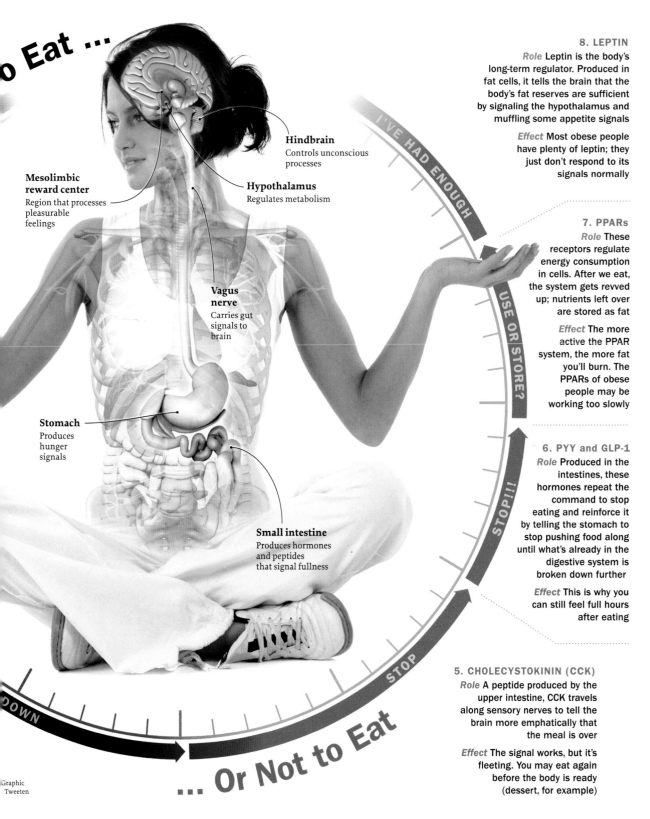

o Eat ...

Mesolimbic reward center
Region that processes pleasurable feelings

Hindbrain
Controls unconscious processes

Hypothalamus
Regulates metabolism

Vagus nerve
Carries gut signals to brain

Stomach
Produces hunger signals

Small intestine
Produces hormones and peptides that signal fullness

I'VE HAD ENOUGH

USE OR STORE?

STOP!!!!

STOP

DOWN

... Or Not to Eat

Graphic
Tweeten

8. LEPTIN
Role Leptin is the body's long-term regulator. Produced in fat cells, it tells the brain that the body's fat reserves are sufficient by signaling the hypothalamus and muffling some appetite signals

Effect Most obese people have plenty of leptin; they just don't respond to its signals normally

7. PPARs
Role These receptors regulate energy consumption in cells. After we eat, the system gets revved up; nutrients left over are stored as fat

Effect The more active the PPAR system, the more fat you'll burn. The PPARs of obese people may be working too slowly

6. PYY and GLP-1
Role Produced in the intestines, these hormones repeat the command to stop eating and reinforce it by telling the stomach to stop pushing food along until what's already in the digestive system is broken down further

Effect This is why you can still feel full hours after eating

5. CHOLECYSTOKININ (CCK)
Role A peptide produced by the upper intestine, CCK travels along sensory nerves to tell the brain more emphatically that the meal is over

Effect The signal works, but it's fleeting. You may eat again before the body is ready (dessert, for example)

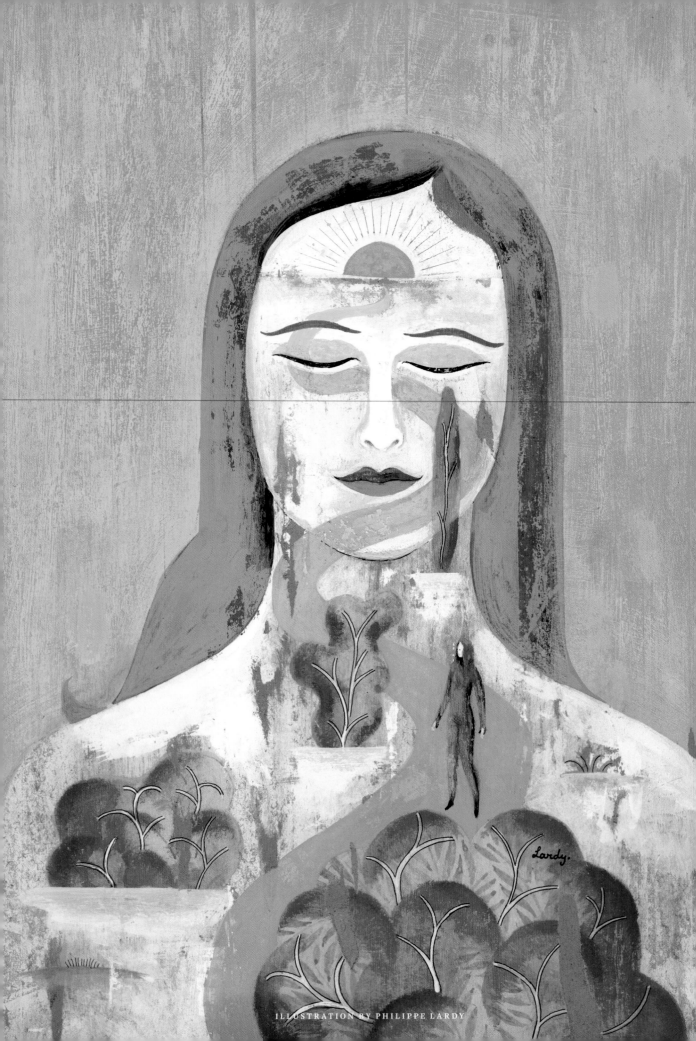

healing

There seems to be no shortage of ways we get sick—but there may be just as many ways we can get ourselves well. A lot of them start with our minds and beliefs

The Power Of Mood

If it seems as though happier people are generally healthier, there's a reason for that: they are. There are powerful links between mind and body—ones we can all put to use

BY DAVID BJERKLIE AND MICHAEL D. LEMONICK

ILL VALVO COULD SENSE THAT something was going very wrong with his health. He had worked for a software-development company in Fairfax, Va., for 10 years following a 22-year hitch with the Air Force, and the pressure was finally too much. "I left to start my own business," says Valvo, "but I could feel that all the stress was having physiological effects."

Sure enough, he was later given a diagnosis of coronary-artery disease and underwent bypass surgery. But after the operation, he spiraled into a severe depression. Eventually, Valvo's physician put him on an antidepressant—which not only relieved the depression but also caused him to think about illness and health in a new way.

"Did my heart operation cause the depression I'm experiencing?" he wrote in an article for a newsletter for Mended Hearts, a support group for heart patients and their families. "Does depression cause heart disease? The answer to both those questions is probably yes."

It may not seem like news these days that an unhealthy mind can lead to an unhealthy body, but not long ago, the mind and the body were seen as two entirely different dimensions of our being. Sure, being sick could make you feel gloomy, but the idea that the system could operate as powerfully in the other direction was viewed as an interesting idea, perhaps, but one without a whole lot of science behind it. All that has changed.

The way we feel emotionally and the way we feel physically are increasingly seen as equal parts of a single whole—and why shouldn't they be? The brain, after all, is only another organ, and it operates on the same biochemical principles as the thyroid or the spleen. Depression represents an imbalance in that operation—one that can kill just as directly as more obviously physical ailments. Each year in the U.S., 30,000 people commit suicide, with the vast majority of cases attributable to depression. But depression's physical toll goes far beyond that. Once you have had a heart attack, for example, your risk of dying from cardiovascular disease is up to six times greater if you also suffer from depression.

The mechanism behind that increased mortality seems obvious: you're depressed because you have a serious illness, and since depressed people smoke or are too lethargic to take their medicine or eat right or exercise, the situation only gets worse. But things aren't that simple. "Even when we take those factors into consideration," says Dr. Dwight Evans, a professor of psychiatry, medicine and neuroscience at the University of Pennsylvania, "depression jumps out as an independent risk factor for heart disease. It may be as bad as cholesterol."

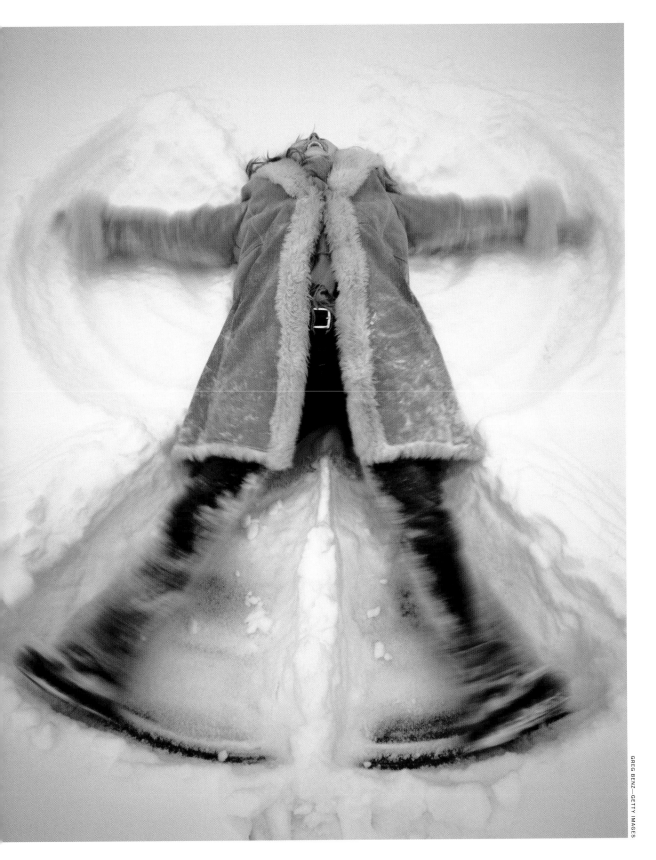

117

Some of the science behind the mind-body link is easy for even nonscientists to understand. When your mind feels terror, the resulting surge of adrenaline makes your stomach churn. When your mind is sexually aroused, the body responds in unmistakable ways. The effect is even more direct with the 60 or so chemicals known as neurotransmitters. Serotonin, for example, circulates everywhere, not only in the brain. "Depression is a systemic disorder," says Evans, "and many of the neurotransmitters that we believe are involved in the pathophysiology of depression have effects throughout the body."

Precisely how these powerful chemicals affect the course of heart disease, cancer and other illnesses isn't well understood, but preliminary research has yielded some tantalizing clues. When serotonin circulates in the bloodstream, for example, it appears to make platelets less sticky and thus less likely to clump in artery-blocking blood clots. For years, heart-attack survivors have been advised to take a children's aspirin daily for clot prevention; drugs like Prozac, which keeps serotonin in circulation, seem to have a similar effect.

Another mechanism may also be at work. It turns out that the heartbeat of a person with depression is unusually steady. That's not necessarily a good thing, says Dr. Dennis Charney, head of mood-and-anxiety-disorders research at the National Institute of Mental

Health (NIMH): "Ideally, your heart rate should be variable—it means your heart can respond appropriately to the different tasks it's called upon to respond to." Yet another possible link between heart disease and depression is a chemical called C-reactive protein (CRP). The liver normally produces CRP in response to an immune-system alarm when the body is infected or injured, and CRP is associated with the inflammation that results. For reasons still unknown, though, depressed individuals, a recent study found, have elevated levels of CRP. And in patients whose arteries have been damaged by the buildup of cholesterol plaques, heightened inflammation may increase the chance that a bit of plaque will break off and shut down an artery.

Diabetes is another illness that worsens with depression. It's well known that 10% of diabetic men and 20% of diabetic women are also depressed, or about twice the rate in the general population. Depressed diabetics are also much more likely than those without depression to suffer complications such as heart disease, nerve damage and blindness.

The obvious cause and effect—having diabetes is depressing—is certainly at play here, but scientists don't think that entirely explains the phenomenon. Somehow, depression appears to make the body less responsive to insulin, the hormone that processes blood sugar—possibly through the action of cortisol, a stress-related hormone that can interfere with insulin sensitivity. Cortisol may also make depressed patients more prone to os-

How Stress Takes Its Toll

Like its more severe cousin depression, ordinary stress is harmful to the body as well as the mind. How it works

1 A STRESS RESPONSE STARTS IN THE BRAIN

When the brain detects a threat, a number of structures, including the hypothalamus, amygdala and pituitary gland, go on alert. They exchange information with one another and then send signaling hormones and nerve impulses to the rest of the body to prepare to fight or flee.

2 THE BODY UNLEASHES A FLOOD OF HORMONES

Adrenal glands react to the alert by releasing adrenaline, which makes the heart pump faster and the lungs work harder to flood the body with oxygen. The adrenal glands

also release extra cortisol and other glucocorticoids, which help the body convert sugars into energy. Nerve cells release norepinephrine, which tenses the muscles and sharpens the senses to prepare for action.

3 THESE HORMONES CAN CAUSE SIGNIFICANT DAMAGE

When the threat passes, epinephrine and norepinephrine levels drop, but if danger comes too often, they can damage the arteries. Chronic low-level stress keeps the glucocorticoids in circulation, leading to a weakened immune system, loss of bone mass, suppression of the reproductive system and memory problems.

4 THE LESSON, IF YOU WANT TO UNDO THAT DAMAGE

Stay calm. There's nothing wrong with the fight-or-flight response when it's needed. But on the subway or in traffic is not the place. Relax; your health depends on it.

teoporosis. Studies by Dr. Philip Gold and Dr. Giovanni Cizza at the NIMH have shown that premenopausal women who are depressed have a much higher rate of bone loss than their nondepressed counterparts, and this disparity increases as women pass through menopause. Cortisol appears to interfere with the ability of the bones to absorb calcium and offset the natural calcium loss that comes with menopause and aging.

Studies have established links between the incidence of depression and several other diseases, including cancer, Parkinson's disease, epilepsy, stroke and Alzheimer's. Parkinson's is caused by the death of cells in the brain that produce the neurotransmitter dopamine. While dopamine is crucial to the control of movement, it's probably a major factor in mood as well. "Depression almost certainly has multiple causes that produce similar symptoms," observes Dr. Bruce Cohen, president of McLean Hospital in Belmont, Mass.

That could explain why drugs that improve serotonin chemistry alone don't always work on depression—and why Parkinson's and depression can feed on each other. Epilepsy, stroke and Alzheimer's, which, like Parkinson's, involve physical alteration of the brain, probably also affect the production and processing of neurotransmitters—not only serotonin and dopamine but also glutamate and norepinephrine, all of which may be involved in different forms of depression.

So can treating depression prevent disease? No, but it can surely help reduce its likelihood. Given that, many

20%
Share of diabetic women who are depressed. Among men, it's 10%

600%
Rise in mortality for heart-attack patients who are also depressed

$50 BILLION
Cost of depression in lost productivity in the U.S. each year

experts hope that physicians will begin to make mental-health assessments a routine part of annual checkups. But that's been proposed before, and it hasn't come easy. "When you only have roughly eight minutes with your primary doctor," says Lydia Lewis, president of the Depression and Bipolar Support Alliance, "it's kind of hard to get into the realm of depression. And when you go to see a specialist, the cardiologist is thinking just about your heart."

So while researchers hold conferences, conduct studies and write scholarly papers, Lewis has some more immediate advice for patients looking to enlist whatever tools are available to help them stay well. "We need to get people to go in and ask these questions of their physicians," she says. Bill Valvo, who learned this lesson more powerfully than most, could not agree more. "I think people are totally unaware of what's going on," he says, "and I'm convinced that education is a key part of what we need to be doing." The essence of that education: cure the mind, and you might just help save the body. ■

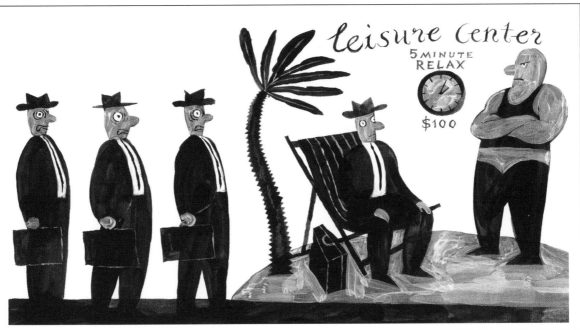

Mind Food
And Other Brain Boosters

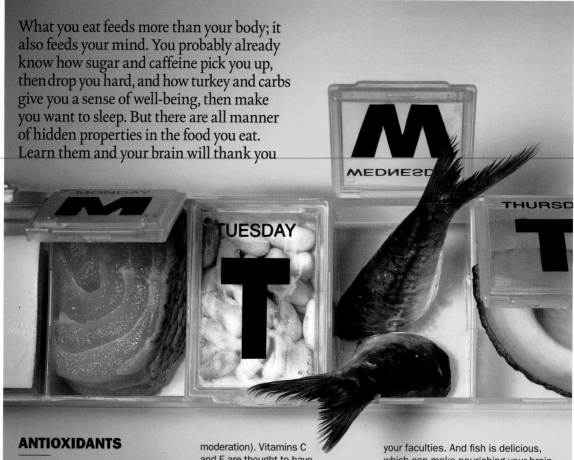

What you eat feeds more than your body; it also feeds your mind. You probably already know how sugar and caffeine pick you up, then drop you hard, and how turkey and carbs give you a sense of well-being, then make you want to sleep. But there are all manner of hidden properties in the food you eat. Learn them and your brain will thank you

ANTIOXIDANTS

FRUITS, VEGETABLES, NUTS AND CHOCOLATE

Oxygen is one of the brain's main fuels, but oxygen can wear it down too—at least the wrong kind can. Common by-products of normal metabolism are so-called free radicals, highly reactive oxygen molecules that lack an electron and can be damaging to healthy tissue. Foods high in what are known as antioxidants can help correct the problem by donating one of their electrons to the radicals, neutralizing their reactivity. Lots of foods are high in antioxidants, notably vegetables and fruits (especially ripe blueberries), as well as chocolate and nuts (though these should be eaten in moderation). Vitamins C and E are thought to have good antioxidant powers, but the best way to get vitamins is in your food.

OMEGA-3

GO FISHING

You've heard it before: Fish is brain food. There's a reason people keep repeating it. While low-fat diets are good for cardiovascular health and weight control, the particular fats in many kinds of fish—known as omega-3 fatty acids—are critical for the growth of the outer membrane of brain cells. Omega-3s are thought to contribute to greater alertness, lower the risk of dementia and generally help you retain your faculties. And fish is delicious, which can make nourishing your brain a treat for your palate.

CAFFEINE AND SUGAR

GO EASY

You feel sharper after you have your coffee or tea in the morning, and a candy bar in the middle of the afternoon does provide an energy bump. But the crash that comes afterward is real. Too much caffeine messes with sleep cycles and heart rate and makes you jumpy; too much sugar leaves you wired. Have coffee, tea and energy drinks only in moderation, and try to opt for the natural sugar in fruit over the refined stuff in candy and soda.

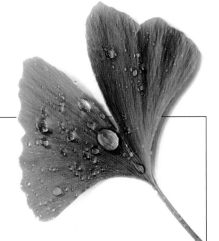

TALKING CURES

TODAY'S TREATMENTS
Most research is focused on the physiology of depression, yet clinicians find that approaches combining medical and psychological treatments are still the most effective. Traditional Freudian therapy is largely gone—and barely missed. Still, doctors do find value in getting patients to probe unconscious roots of their problems. Newer techniques like cognitive therapy are more direct, teaching patients to recognize destructive patterns and develop practical steps to change them.

ON THE HORIZON
Meditation, mindfulness training and biofeedback have long been championed as proven stress relievers. Now proponents believe these techniques may also provide relief for people with depression by lowering levels of cortisol, a stress hormone.

ALTERNATIVE REMEDIES

TODAY'S TREATMENTS
Many patients help themselves to over-the-counter aids, from St.-John's-wort to ginkgo biloba and soybean extracts. But herbs, like prescription drugs, can have side effects, and researchers are investigating their efficacy. The popular supplement DHEA, for example, has been linked to an increased risk of cancer.

ON THE HORIZON
Probiotics are bacteria, like the kind found in yogurt, that have health benefits. Other strains are being marketed in foods and supplements to help treat intestinal and urinary problems, eczema and more.

DRUGS

TODAY'S TREATMENTS
Most antidepressants work by tweaking levels of neurotransmitters, the chemicals that carry signals between neurons. By preventing excess neurotransmitters from being reabsorbed too quickly, they leave some in circulation and improve mood. Another class of drugs, monoamine oxidase inhibitors, can be effective but can also produce dangerous side effects. Anticonvulsives and antipsychotics are prescribed for conditions including bipolar disorder and schizophrenia. Stimulants have their uses as well, principally in treating attention-deficit/hyperactivity disorder.

ON THE HORIZON
Researchers are exploring two molecules, gaba and glutamate, that are responsible for 90% of signaling in the brain. The trick would be to fine-tune their levels to relieve depression but not affect normal functions. Other targets of drug studies: testosterone (a skin patch proved effective in a clinical trial for men), the stress hormone cortisol, a chemical called substance P (found in pain pathways), compounds called CRF antagonists, and the dynorphins— the evil twins of feel-good endorphins. ■

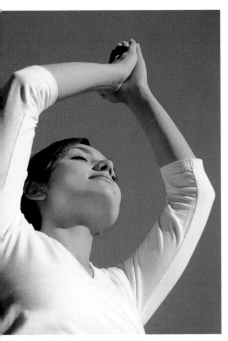

ELECTRICAL AND MAGNETIC THERAPIES

TODAY'S TREATMENTS
Electroshock therapy, despite its unsavory reputation, can actually be quite effective, especially for patients who don't respond to drugs and seniors for whom drug interactions pose problems. The treatment today uses a small current to trigger a mild seizure—a rhythmic firing of neurons—that can push a depressed brain out of its rut.

ON THE HORIZON
Researchers have been exploring a technique called repetitive transcranial magnetic stimulation, which administers a series of magnetic pulses to the head. These induce a low-level electrical current in neurons that seems to reset the brain and improve mood. How does it work? No one is exactly certain, but the best hypothesis is that when the pulse is applied to the cortex—a higher region of the brain—it helps restore synchrony with lower regions like the limbic area. Scientists liken the results to a computer after rebooting.

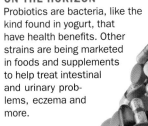

The Biology Of Belief

Atheists and believers may argue about religion, but one thing seems clear: having faith can improve your health. The next debate is inevitable: Why?

By Jeffrey Kluger

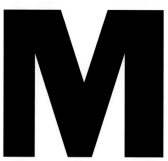

MOST FOLKS PROBABLY couldn't locate their parietal lobe with a map and a compass. For the record, it's at the top of your head—aft of the frontal lobe, fore of the occipital lobe, north of the temporal lobe. What makes the parietal lobe special is not where it lives but what it does—particularly concerning matters of faith.

If you've ever prayed so hard that you've lost all sense of a larger world outside yourself, that's your parietal lobe at work. If you've ever meditated so deeply that you'd swear the very boundaries of your body had dissolved, that's your parietal too. There are other regions responsible for making your brain the spiritual amusement park it can be: your thalamus plays a role, as do your frontal lobes. But it's your parietal lobe—a central mass of tissue that processes sensory input—that may have the most transporting effect.

Needy creatures that we are, we put the brain's spiritual centers to use all the time. We pray for peace; we meditate for serenity; we chant for wealth. We travel to Lourdes in search of a miracle; we go to Mecca to show our devotion; we eat hallucinogenic mushrooms to attain transcendent vision and gather in church basements to achieve its sober opposite. But there is nothing we pray—or chant or meditate—for more than health.

Health, by definition, is the sine qua non of everything else. If you're dead, serenity is academic. So we convince ourselves that while our medicine is strong and our doctors are wise, our prayers may heal us too.

Here's what's surprising: a growing body of scientific evidence suggests that faith may indeed bring us health. People who attend religious services do have a lower risk of dying in any given year than people who don't attend. People who believe in a loving God fare better after a diagnosis of illness than people who believe in a punitive God. No less a killer than AIDS will back off at least a bit when it's hit with a double-barreled blast of belief. "Even accounting for medications," says Dr. Gail Ironson, a professor of psychiatry and psychology at the University of Miami who studies HIV and religious belief, "spirituality predicts for better disease control."

It's hard not to be impressed by findings like that, but a skeptic will say there's nothing remarkable—much less spiritual—about them. You live longer if you go to church because you're there for the cholesterol-screening drive and the visiting-nurse service. Your viral load goes down when you include spirituality in your fight against HIV because your levels of cortisol—a stress hormone—go down first. "Science doesn't deal

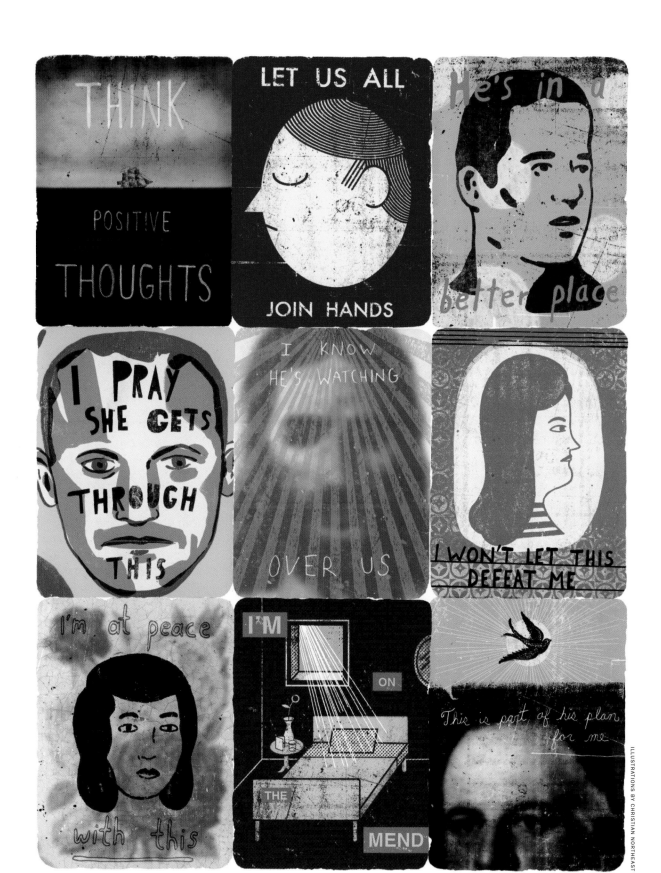

in supernatural explanations," says Richard Sloan, a professor of behavioral medicine at Columbia University Medical Center and the author of *Blind Faith: The Unholy Alliance of Religion and Medicine.* "Religion and science address different concerns."

That's undeniably true—up to a point. But it's also true that our brains and bodies contain an awful lot of spiritual wiring. Even if there's a scientific explanation for every strand of it, that doesn't mean we can't put it to powerful use. And if one of those uses can make us well, shouldn't we take advantage of it? Says Dr. Andrew Newberg, a professor of radiology, psychology and religious studies at the University of Pennsylvania and the co-founder of Penn's Center for Spirituality and the Mind: "The way the brain works is so compatible with religion and spirituality that we're going to be enmeshed in both for a long time."

Enmeshed in the brain is as good a way as any to describe Newberg's work of the past 15 years. The author of four books, including *How God Changes Your Brain,* he has looked more closely than most at how our spiritual data-processing center works, conducting various types of brain scans on more than 100 people, all in different kinds of worshipful or contemplative states. Over time, Newberg and his team have come to recognize just which parts of the brain light up during just which experiences.

When people engage in prayer, it's the frontal lobes that take the lead; that makes sense, since they govern focus and concentration. During very deep prayer, the parietal lobe powers down, which is what allows us to experience that transcendent sense of having loosed our earthly moorings. The frontal lobes go quieter when worshippers are involved in the singular activity of speaking in tongues—which jibes nicely with the

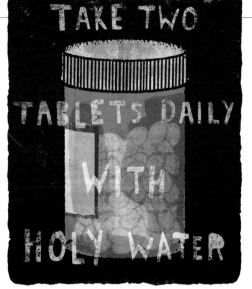

speakers' subjective experience that they are not in control of what they're saying.

Pray and meditate enough, and some changes in the brain become permanent. Long-term meditators—those with 15 years of practice or more—appear to have thicker frontal lobes than nonmeditators. People who describe themselves as highly spiritual tend to exhibit an asymmetry in the thalamus—a feature that other people can develop after just eight weeks of training in meditation skills. "It may be that some people have fundamental asymmetry [in the thalamus] to begin with," Newberg says, "and that leads them down this path, which changes the brain further."

No matter what explains the shape of the brain, it can pay dividends. For one thing, better-functioning frontal lobes help boost memory. In one study, Newberg scanned the brains of people who complained of poor recall before they underwent meditation training, then scanned them again after. As the lobes bulked up, memory improved.

Faith and health overlap in other ways too. Take fasting. One of the staples of both traditional wellness protocols and traditional religious rituals is the cleansing fast, which is said to purge toxins in the first case and purge sins or serve other pious ends in the second. Done right, these fasts may lead to a state of clarity and even euphoria. This, in turn, can give practitioners the blissful sense that whether the goal of the food restriction is health or spiritual insight, it's being achieved. Maybe it is, but there's also chemical legerdemain at work.

The brain is a very energy-intensive organ, one that requires a lot of calories to keep running. When food intake is cut, the liver steps into the breach, producing glucose and sending it throughout the body—always making sure the brain gets a particularly generous help-

---

PLACEBO POWER **When Parkinson's patients underwent sham surgery said to boost dopamine, levels of the neurotransmitter actually increased.** ALL TIED UP **Complications occurred in 52% of heart-bypass patients who received intercessory prayer and 51% who didn't— a statistical wash.** HELPER'S HIGH **Stress goes down more among parishioners who offer support than among those who receive it.**

EXTENDING TIME **Church attendance may add two to three years of life. Exercise may add three to five, and statin therapy 2.4 to 3.5.**

ing. The liver's reserve lasts only about 24 hours, after which cells begin breaking down the body's fats and proteins—essentially living off the land. As this happens, the composition of the blood—including hormones, neurotransmitters and metabolic by-products—changes. Throw this much loopy chemistry at a sensitive machine like the brain, and it's likely to go on the blink. "There are very real changes that occur in the body very rapidly that might explain the clarity during fasting," says Dr. Catherine Gordon, an endocrinologist at Children's Hospital in Boston. "The brain is in a different state, even during a short-term fast." Biologically, that's not good, but the light-headed sense of peace, albeit brief, that comes with it reinforces the fast and rewards you for engaging in it all the same.

For most believers, the element of religious life that intersects most naturally with health is prayer. Very serious theologians believe in the power of so-called intercessory prayer to heal the sick, and some very serious scientists have looked at it too: more than 6,000 studies on the topic have been published just since 2000.

As long ago as 1872, Francis Galton, the man behind eugenics and fingerprinting, reckoned that monarchs should live longer than the rest of us, since millions of people pray for the health of their King or Queen every day. His research showed just the opposite—no surprise, perhaps, given the rich diet and extensive leisure that royal families enjoy. An oft discussed 1988 study by cardiologist Randolph Byrd of San Francisco General Hospital took a more rigorous look at the same question and found that heart patients who were prayed for fared better than those who were not. But a larger study in 2005 by cardiologist Herbert Benson at Harvard University challenged that finding, reporting that complications occurred in 52% of heart-bypass patients who received intercessory prayer and 51% of those who didn't—essentially a tie.

Such findings don't typically dissuade believers—not unexpectedly, perhaps, considering the centrality of prayer to faith. But there is one thing on which both camps agree: when you're setting up your study, it matters a great deal whether subjects know they're being prayed for. Give them even a hint as to whether they're in the prayer group or a control group, and the famed placebo effect can blow your data to bits.

First described in medical literature in the 1780s, the placebo effect can work all manner of curative magic against all manner of ills. Give a patient a sugar pill but call it an analgesic, and pain may actually go away. Parkinson's-disease patients who underwent a sham surgery that they were told would boost the low dopamine levels responsible for their symptoms actually experienced a dopamine bump. "The brain appears to be able to target the placebo effect in a variety of ways," says Newberg. There's no science proving that the intercessions of others will make you well. But it probably does no harm—and in fact probably helps—to know that people are sending prayers your way.

If the value of being prayed for continues to spark arguments, the value of praying in a group—in a church or a synagogue or another house of worship—is a more settled matter. Social demographer Robert Hummer of the University of Texas has been following a population of subjects since 1992, and his results are hard to argue with. Those who never attend religious services have twice the risk of dying over the next eight years as people who attend once a week. People who fall somewhere between no churchgoing and weekly churchgoing also

6,000

Number of studies on remote prayer since 2000. One of the first was in 1872; it tested the idea that monarchs should have long lives, since millions of people pray for their health

fall somewhere between in terms of mortality.

Other studies show similar results, and while investigators haven't teased out all the variables at work in this phenomenon, some of the factors are no surprise. "People embedded in religious communities are more likely to rely on one another for friendship, support, rides to doctor's appointments," says Hummer.

That's not all, however, and even hard scientists concede that there's a constellation of other variables at work that are far tougher to measure. "Religious belief is not just a mind question but involves the commitment of one's body as well," says Ted Kaptchuk, a professor of medicine at Harvard Medical School. "The sensory organs, tastes, smells, sounds, music, the architecture of religious buildings [are involved]." Just as the mere act of coming into a hospital exposes a patient to sights and smells that can prime the brain and body for healing, so may the act of walking into a house of worship.

Neal Krause, a sociologist and public-health expert at the University of Michigan, has tried to quantify some of those more amorphous variables in a longitudinal study of 1,500 people that he has been conducting since 1997. He has focused particularly on how regular churchgoers weather economic downturns as well as the stresses and health woes that go along with them. Not surprisingly, he has found that parishioners benefit when they receive social support from their church. And he has discovered that those people who give help fare even better than those who receive it—a pillar of religious belief if ever there was one. He has also found that people who maintain a sense of gratitude for what's going right in their lives have a reduced incidence of depression, which is itself a predictor of health.

African-American churches have been especially good at maximizing the connection between faith and health. Earlier in American history, churches were the only institutions American blacks had the freedom to establish and run themselves, and they thus became deeply embedded in the culture. "The black church is a different institution than the synagogue or mosque or even the white church," says Ken Resnicow, a professor of health and behavior education at the University of Michigan School of Public Health. "It is the center of spiritual, community and political life."

Given the generally higher incidence of obesity, hypertension and other lifestyle ills among African Americans, the church is in a powerful position to do a lot of good. In the 1990s, Marci Campbell, a professor of nutrition at the University of North Carolina, helped launch a four-year trial called North Carolina Black Churches United for Better Health. The project signed up 50 churches with the goal of helping the 2,500 parishioners eat better, exercise more and generally improve their fitness. The measures taken included such straightfor-

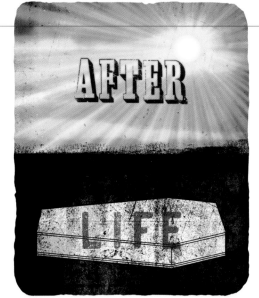

ward strategies as having pastors preach health in their sermons and getting churches to serve healthier foods at community events. The program was so successful that it has been renamed the Body and Soul project and rolled out nationally—complete with literature, DVDs and cookbooks—in collaboration with the National Cancer Institute and the American Cancer Society.

Many scientists and theologians who study all these matters advocate a system in which both pastoral and medical care are offered as parts of a whole—and that can work particularly well not just in the church but in a doctor's office or hospital too. If a woman given a diagnosis of breast cancer is already offered the services of an oncologist, a psychologist and a reconstructive surgeon, why shouldn't her doctor discuss her religious needs with her and include a pastor in the mix if that would help?

While churches are growing increasingly willing to accept the assistance of health-care experts, doctors and hospitals have been slower to seek out the help of spiritual counselors. The fear has long been that patients aren't interested in asking such spiritually intimate questions of their doctors, and the doctors, for their part, would be uncomfortable answering them. But this turns out not to be true. When psychologist Jean Kristeller of Indiana State University conducted a survey of oncologists, she found that a large proportion of them did feel it was appropriate to talk about spiritual issues with patients and to offer a referral if they weren't equipped to answer questions themselves. They didn't do so simply because they didn't know how to raise the topic and feared giving offense. When patients were asked, they insisted that they'd welcome such a conversation but that their doctors had never initiated one.

Kristeller, who had participated in earlier work exploring how physicians could help their patients quit

---

HOW RELIGIONS VIEW THE BEYOND
Medicine and religion both can be seen as responses to the prospect of death. Science is quiet on a possible afterlife; religious practices may be shaped by it

BUDDHISM
Though specific beliefs vary by sect, Buddhists hold fast to the doctrine of reincarnation, ending only in the final liberation known as Nirvana

CHRISTIANITY
The vast majority of Christians believe in the concept of heaven and hell. Your destination is believed to depend on your deeds and faith during life

smoking, recalled a short, five- to seven-minute conversation that the leader of a study had devised to help doctors address that problem. The recommended dialogue conformed to what's known as patient-centered care—a clinical way of saying doctors should ask questions, then clam up and listen to the answers. In the case of smoking, they were advised merely to make their concern known to patients, then ask them if they'd ever tried to quit before. Depending on how that first question was received, doctors could ask when those earlier attempts were made, whether the patients would be interested in trying again and, most important, if it was all right to follow up on the conversation in the future. "The more patient-centered the conversations were, the more impact they had," Kristeller says.

The success of that approach led her to develop a similar guide for doctors who want to discuss religious questions with cancer patients. The approach has not yet been tested in any large-scale studies, but in the smaller surveys Kristeller has conducted, it has been a success: up to 90% of the patients whose doctors approached them in this way were not offended by the overture, and 75% said it was very helpful. Within as little as three weeks, the people in that group reported reduced feelings of depression, an improved quality of life and a greater sense that their doctors cared about them.

Even doctors who aren't familiar with Kristeller's script are finding it easier to combine spiritual care and medical care. HealthCare Chaplaincy is an organization of Christian, Jewish, Muslim and Zen Buddhist board-certified chaplains affiliated with more than a dozen hospitals and clinics in the New York City area. The group routinely provides pastoral care to patients as part of the total package of treatment. The chaplains, like doctors, have a caseload of patients they visit on their rounds, taking what amounts to a spiritual history

94%

Share of patients who say it is all right for doctors to ask them about their religious beliefs and discuss the role faith may play in their recovery. Doctors don't ask for fear of giving offense

and either offering counseling on their own or referring patients to others. The Rev. Walter Smith, president and CEO of the chaplaincy and an end-of-life specialist, sees what his group offers as a health-care product—one that is not limited to believers.

"When people say, 'I'm not sure you can help because I'm not very religious,'" Smith explains, "the chaplains say, 'That's not a problem. Can I sit down and engage you in conversation?'"

Patients who say yes often find themselves exploring what they consider secular questions that touch on such primal matters of life and death, they might as well be spiritual ones. The chaplains can also refer patients to other care providers, such as social workers, psychologists and guided-imagery specialists. "People say you tell the truth to your doctor, your priest and your funeral director," says Smith, "because these people matter at the end." It's that truth—or at least a path to it—that chaplains seek to provide.

Smith's group is slowly expanding, hoping to go national, and even the most literal-minded scientists have no quarrel with such a development. Says Sloan, the author of *Blind Faith:* "I think that a chaplain's job is to explore the patient's values and help the patient come to some decision. I think that's absolutely right."

Sloan's view is catching on. Few people think of religion as an alternative to medicine. The frontline tools of an emergency room will always be splints and sutures, and well-applied medicine along with smart prevention will always be the most effective way to stay well. Still, if the U.S.'s expanding health-care emergency has taught us anything, it's that we can't afford to be choosy about where we look for answers. Doctors, patients and pastors battling disease already know that help comes in a whole lot of forms. It's the result, not the source, that counts the most. ∎

HINDUISM
Like Buddhists, Hindus believe in reincarnation and karma, with your status in your next life depending on how you conduct yourself in this one

ISLAM
Similar to Christians, Muslims believe in a day of judgment in the afterlife, when the dead will be divided between paradise and damnation

JUDAISM
Jewish texts have little to say about a possible afterlife, placing greater emphasis on virtuous actions in this life, not the one to come

The Puzzle Of Love

Romance and sex are all about chemistry—and that's not just a metaphor. A process that starts in the brain cascades through the body, turning simple biology into bliss

BY JEFFREY KLUGER
AND MICHAEL D. LEMONICK

O F ALL THE SPLENDIDLY RIdiculous, transcendently fulfilling things humans do, it's sex that most confounds understanding. What in the world are we doing? Why in the world are we so consumed by it? The impulse to procreate may lie at the heart of sex, but like the impulse to nourish ourselves, it is merely the starting point for an astonishingly varied banquet. Bursting from our sexual center is a whole spangle of other things—art, song, romance, obsession, rapture, sorrow, companionship, love, even violence and criminality—all playing an enormous role in everything from our physical and emotional health to our very life spans.

Why should this be so? Did nature simply overload us in the mating department, hot-wiring us for the sex that is so central to the survival of the species—and never mind the sometimes sloppy consequences? Or is there something smarter and subtler at work, some larger interplay among sexuality, life and what it means to be human?

No matter how lust is triggered, sex, like eating or sleeping, is ultimately biochemical, governed by hormones, neurotransmitters and other substances that interact in complicated ways to create the familiar sensations of desire, arousal and orgasm. Over the past decade or two, scientists have identified many of the pieces of this puzzle. For both men and women, it clearly involves testosterone, along with other hormones, including estrogen and oxytocin, and brain chemicals such as dopamine, serotonin and norepinephrine. Scientists have also learned that the old notion that 90% of sex is in the mind is literally true: the parts of the brain involved in sexual response include, at the very least, the sensory vagus nerves, the midbrain reticular formation, the basal ganglia, the anterior insula cortex, the amygdala, the cerebellum and the hypothalamus.

Researchers are still struggling to understand how these pieces fit together and how they might be different for men and women. It's not clear which chemicals of desire are unleashed and under which circumstances, for example, because setting and mood, as women know better than men, can make all the difference between arousal and annoyance.

Dr. Jennifer Berman, a urologist and director of the Female Sexual Medicine Center at UCLA, says, "Women experience desire as a result of context—how they feel about themselves and their partner, how safe they feel, their closeness and their attachment." Men, says Berman, "tend to be more visually directed and stimulated than women are." Thus *Playboy* and Hooters

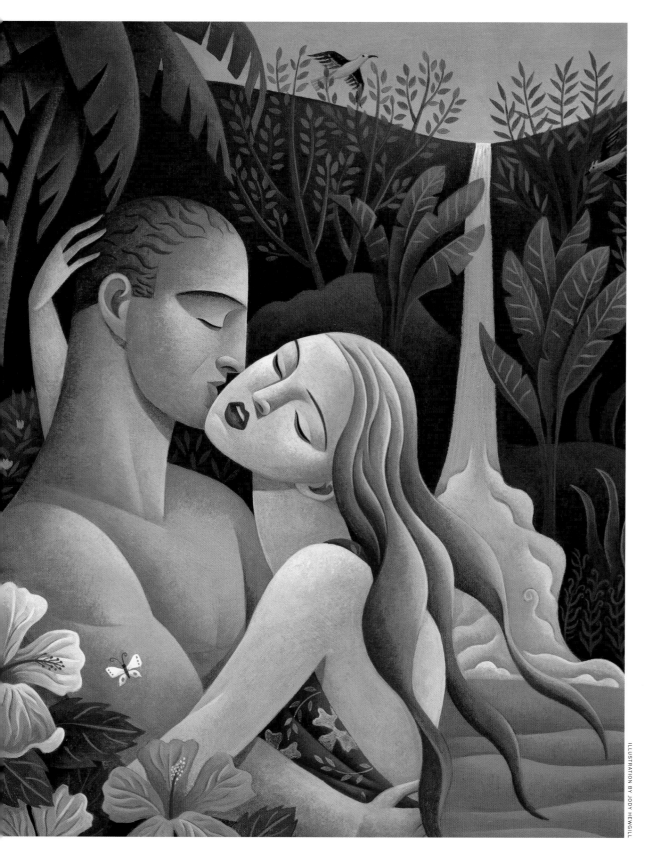

and the estimated $10 billion–a–year, mainly male-oriented pornography industry.

But the reasons for that difference may be as much cultural as they are physiological. Dr. Julia Heiman, a psychologist and director of the Reproductive and Sexual Medicine Clinic at the University of Washington Medical School, is one of a growing number of researchers who think it's misguided to see men as simple and linear and women as complex and circular. "I don't think we've taken the time to talk to men about what desire is," she says. "If they are emotional about their sexuality, they don't feel in step with other men."

Women who don't fit stereotypes don't fare much better, says Jim Pfaus, a psychologist at Concordia University in Montreal who studies behavioral neurobiology. "What is a woman who expresses arousal in response to blatantly visual sexual cues? I hope we've moved beyond calling her a slut while calling a man who does the same a stud." But the cultural prejudice behind those labels persists, he says.

Research by Meredith Chivers at the Center for Addiction and Mental Health, affiliated with the University of Toronto, shows that women do respond to sexy visual stimuli. In fact, in one study, Chivers found that women show physical signs of arousal in response to a wider variety of images (including films of bonobo chimps mating) than men do. But unlike in men, this physical arousal is not closely paired with a subjective feeling of being turned on. In short, physical arousal for women can come before or even in the absence of conscious desire—doubtless a source of much confusion between the sexes.

But while arousal and desire are intimately intertwined and probably involve all sorts of feedback between brain and genitalia, at least some of the underlying biochemistry is becoming clear. If there's one substance that makes it possible for any of us to get turned on in the first place, testosterone is probably it. "When testosterone is gone," says Berman, "for whatever reason—aging, medication—men experience erection and libido problems." Restore the testosterone, and you usually fix those problems.

Women too seem to have problems getting interested in sex when their testosterone levels are too low. Says Dr.

The hormone oxytocin is often called the cuddle chemical. It plays a vital role in nursing and soars when either parent holds a new baby. It may even rise when couples hold hands, hug or watch a romantic movie

Alan Altman, a specialist in menopause and sexuality at Harvard Medical School: "When women are having normal menstrual cycles in their prime reproductive ages, their ovaries make two times more testosterone than estrogen." A few days before ovulation, sexual desire peaks, triggered by surging levels of testosterone, along with other hormones, including progesterone and estrogen.

For women, at least, estrogen may also be crucial. "Give estrogen to women with decreased desire," says Pfaus, "and you don't restore desire. Give them testosterone alone, and you get a little increase in desire. Give them estrogen and testosterone together, and you get a whopping increase."

Both testosterone and estrogen trigger desire by stimulating the release of neurotransmitters in the brain. The most important of these for the feeling we call desire seems to be dopamine. Dopamine is at least partly responsible for making external stimuli arousing. Another neurotransmitter almost certainly involved in the biochemistry of desire is serotonin, which, like dopamine, plays a role in feelings of satisfaction.

Desire, of course, is only part of the procreative equation. So are feelings of tenderness and intimacy, and these too have chemical roots. Endocrinologists have known for years that oxytocin, released by the pituitary gland, ovaries and testes, helps trigger childbirth contractions, milk production during nursing and the pelvic shudders women experience during orgasm (and possibly the contractions during male orgasm as well). The hormone is believed to play a vital role in mother-child bonding and may do the same for new fathers: oxytocin surges when a new dad holds his baby.

WHERE OUR SEX DRIVE COMES FROM

Dopamine

This is probably the most important neurotransmitter involved in desire. Dopamine-producing neurons in the brain color our perception of the world. In the case of sex, it creates what we experience as a sexy mood. Dopamine also helps us feel pleasure.

Serotonin

Produced in the midbrain and brain stem, this neurotransmitter creates feelings of satisfaction, including those experienced after orgasm. Serotonin can increase desire, but paradoxically, serotonin-boosting drugs like Prozac can inhibit orgasm.

Love, Visualized

You know how you feel when you look at a picture of the person you love. Here's what's going on inside your head

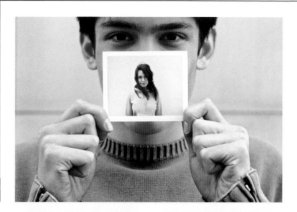

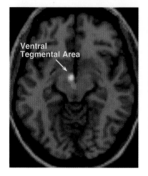

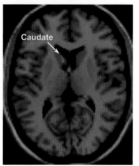

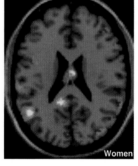

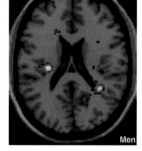

One brain region that grows more active in lovers is the ventral tegmental area, where dopamine neurons are produced and sent to other regions, including the nearby caudate

The caudate nucleus lights up at the same time. This region produces dopamine and plays a role in the brain's reward and motivation systems, which reinforce good feelings

It's hardly a secret that men and women behave differently in romantic situations, but these images make those distinctions stark. Scans reveal that women exposed to romantic triggers show more activity in regions that process attention, emotion and recall. Men, by contrast, are more active in areas associated with the integration of visual stimuli and sexual arousal

Some researchers go so far as to think of oxytocin as the cuddle chemical. Preliminary studies by psychiatrist Kathleen Light at the University of North Carolina have found that oxytocin levels rise after couples hold hands, hug or watch romantic movies. It also may be what makes you want to stay the night with your partner, even after sex.

Another, newly identified substance that has captured Pfaus' interest is alpha melanocyte polypeptide, also known as melanocyte-stimulating hormone. In clinical trials, this pituitary hormone had the dual effect of giving men erections and heightening their interest in sex. "It's astonishing that you have a little peptide that has such a big, specific effect," he says.

Like all other researchers who work to deconstruct sex this way, Pfaus is fascinated by its sheer complexity, and we will surely come to understand more and more. But that understanding could come at a price. We all experience attraction and sexual desire as a thrilling ride and a delightful mystery, far removed from the clinical business of glands and hormones and peptide chemistry. If scientists continue to be at least a little mystified by it all, at least some of that wonder will remain intact. ∎

Epinephrine/Norepinephrine

The pounding heart, increased blood pressure and accelerated respiration that occur during sexual and romantic stimulation are the handiwork of these neurotransmitters. Found in the adrenal glands (above the kidneys), spinal cord and brain, the chemicals play a critical role in facilitating arousal and orgasm.

Testosterone and Estrogen

Testosterone is produced in the testes and ovaries, though it is quickly converted to estrogen in women. When testosterone is low, both sexes experience diminished libido. Estrogen is produced in the ovaries and brain. It stimulates desire in women—and maybe men—possibly by boosting dopamine.

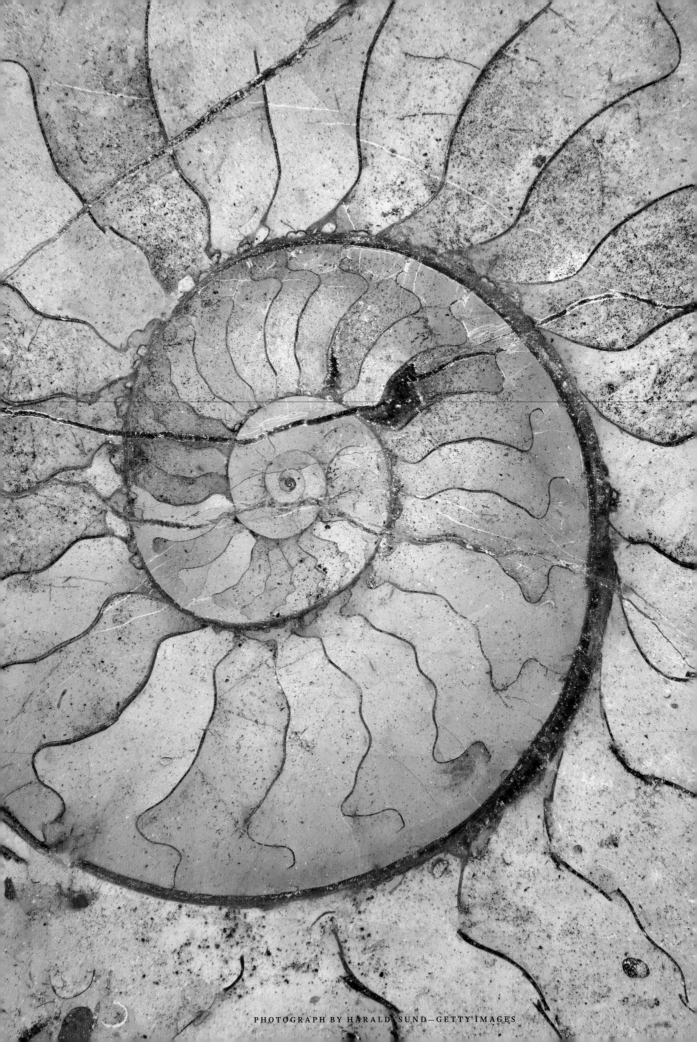

evolution

The brain has always been a work in progress. It grows steadily more complex over the lifetime of a species—and of an individual

From Cells To Beasts To All of Us

Humans are hardly the only animals with brains, but ours are surely the most complex. It took a long time—and a whole lot of evolving—to get where we are

By Carl Zimmer

BETWEEN OUR EARS IS A MARvel of biology. The human brain is made up of billions of neurons woven together in trillions of connections. It allows us to do things no other species can do: understand language, remember events that happened decades ago and make plans for long after we're dead. Such a reasoning machine does not seem to be the kind of thing you could manufacture overnight, and indeed, the human brain has been long in the making. By studying fossils and genes as well as other animals, biologists have been reconstructing its 700 million–year saga.

The story of the brain starts before brains even existed. Animals evolved from single-cell ancestors; studies of DNA reveal that our closest living single-cell relatives are pond-dwelling organisms called choanoflagellates. To get clues to what that long-ago ancestor was like, scientists in 2008 sequenced the entire genome of a choanoflagellate. They discovered that this otherwise unremarkable creature has some genes that had previously been known to exist only in the neurons of far more sophisticated animals.

For example, when young neurons in animals move through the brain to find their final locations, they switch on a gene called reelin, which triggers the production of a protein that helps guide them; choanoflagellates turn out to have a reelin gene too. Neurons make receptors to grab signaling molecules from other parts of the body; choanoflagellates make the same kind of receptors. In order to produce electric pulses, neurons open up specialized channels to let charged calcium atoms flow across their membranes; choanoflagellates are the first nonanimals ever found that have the same kinds of calcium channels. In other words, some of the building blocks of our brains—the genes that would be essential for constructing and operating neurons—already existed in single-cell creatures some 700 million years ago. That's not to say that a creature without a brain had much use for genes that guide the growth of one. Rather, back then the genes had other functions, just as they do in choanoflagellates today. But they can be traced back to that early ancestor all the same.

The earliest animals to evolve from single-cell organisms were probably brainless. One of the oldest lineages of living animals, the sponges, have no neurons. They are essentially clumps of cells anchored to the seafloor, filtering water to trap bits of food. Such bodies are not terribly substantial, yet sponges managed to leave the oldest known animal traces in the

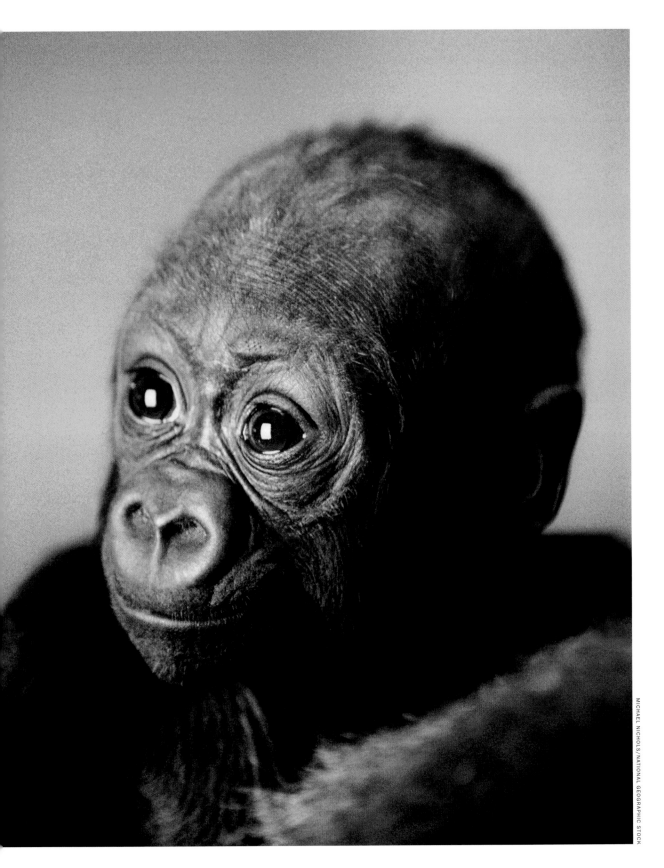

fossil record, dating back 635 million years. Incredibly, even in these simple creatures there are foreshadowings of our brains.

Sponges start life as larvae that drift through the water in search of a place to settle down. Some of the cells on the surface of the larvae, called globular cells, develop a deep pit, out of which grows a long hair. Some studies hint that globular cells sense changes in the movement of water around the larva, which may signal it to settle down to the seafloor. In 2008, Bernard Degnan, a biologist at the University of Queensland in Australia, and his colleagues analyzed the network of genes that guides the development of globular cells. They discovered that each of the genes is closely related to a gene that guides the development of neurons in more complex creatures. Meanwhile, Ken Kosik of the University of California at Santa Barbara has been examining some of the proteins that act as scaffolding inside globular cells. Protein for protein, they show an uncanny resemblance to the scaffolding inside the swellings that neurons use to connect to other neurons, known as synapses. This research powerfully suggests that our neurons evolved from sensory cells like globular cells in sponges.

Aside from sponges, just about all the millions of living animal species have at least rudimentary nervous systems. And complexity aside, those nervous

systems operate in remarkably similar ways. They all generate signals with pulses of electric charge that move from one end of a neuron to the other. They all transmit the signal from neuron to neuron through synapses, using the same neurotransmitters to ferry the information along. And all animals with a nervous system, from us all the way down to jellyfish, use related genes to build neurons.

Together, all this evidence strongly supports the hypothesis that animals inherited their nervous systems from a common ancestor. But the fact that we share ancestral roots does not mean that we follow the same developmental paths. In each lineage, nervous systems evolved in unique directions. Jellyfish, for example, evolved a ring of neurons that encircles their bell-shaped main body. Instead of a single brain, they have clumps of neurons spaced regularly around the ring. In our own ancestors, the nervous system evolved into a very different arrangement. Our system—and the one found in all mammals, birds, reptiles, amphibians and fish—is centered on a large brain in the head and a spinal cord running down the back.

To study how this configuration first evolved, biologists examine some of the closest invertebrate relatives of vertebrates. These creatures, known as lancelets, look like tiny headless sardines. Like us, they have a spinal cord running down their back. The front end of

The Long March Through Time

Our brains started humbly and developed very slowly. It took eons—about 700 million years—to grow the brains we have

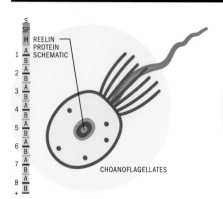

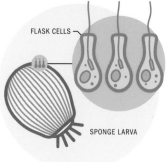

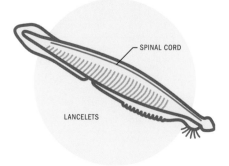

CHOANOFLAGELLATES
No brain in this 700 million–year–old one-celled organism, but what it does have is a gene called reelin, which in later, higher animals helps guide the growth of neurons

SPONGE LARVAE
Sponges, which emerged 635 million years ago, have cells that sense the motion of water. The proteins and genes that guide the cells are similar to those related to neurons

LANCELETS
Invertebrates with many features of vertebrates, they were among the first to develop a body architecture in which the brain sits atop a spine. Their brain is little more than a tiny swelling

their spinal cord is a barely swollen tip. It's not much to look at, but on the lancelet's modest scale, it passes for a brain. What's more, scientists have uncovered a lot of evidence indicating that the earliest vertebrate brains were all very similar. For example, biologists have identified genes that switch on when a lancelet's nerve cord starts to develop. These genes make proteins that mark the front, middle and rear of the nerve cord's tip. The same genes switch on in the same order during the development of our own brains.

The oldest evidence of a true vertebrate nervous system is a cache of hundreds of 535 million–year–old fossils uncovered over the past decade in China. These fossils belong to a tiny fishlike creature called Haikouichthys. Measuring about an inch long, it had many hallmarks of living vertebrates, including two dark spots at the front of its body that appear to be simple eyes. Haikouichthys also had holes on the side of its head where sound-sensitive nerves probably grew and another cavity up front that paleontologists suspect was a nostril. None of these structures allow anything like the fully developed senses we enjoy, but they did provide various ways for the Haikouichthys to recognize—and interact with—its world. Even such rudimentary signals require some central processor to read and interpret them, and the animal's head does contain a mass of cartilage surrounding a small brain.

Over the next 100 million years, humble Haikouichthys–like creatures evolved into the biggest animals in the world. Many of the major features of our nervous systems developed during this transition. Fossils show that as the bodies of fish became longer, their neurons

As primates began to rely more on vision than on scent to find food, the regions of their brains that processed signals from the nose shrank, while those that processed signals from the eyes grew dramatically

did as well. This was made possible by the evolution of myelin, an oily sleeve for neurons that acts like insulation around a wire, preventing the loss of electric signal over long distances. The growing neurons of fish began to supply the brain with information from larger sense organs, and new motor neurons allowed fish to steer their bodies in complex ways.

Controlling those neurons was an increasingly elaborate brain. The brain evolved into three distinct regions, which can still be seen in the brains of all living vertebrates today: the cerebellum, the optic tectum and the cerebrum. Each of these regions took on different functions. The cerebellum, located at the base of the brain, is especially important for balance. People who suffer damage to their cerebellum have trouble walking. Fish use their cerebellum to stay balanced in

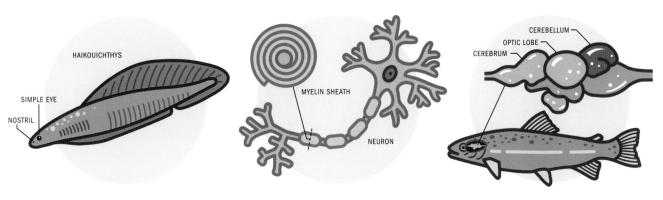

HAIKOUICHTHYS
Barely an inch long, the 535 million–year–old fishlike creature was the first true vertebrate with a nervous system. It had what appear to be primitive eyes, ears and nose, as well as a tiny brain

THE EVOLUTION OF MYELIN
A fatty sheath around nerves, myelin acts like insulation around a wire. Its appearance allowed brains and nervous systems to grow more complex, without the signals getting crossed

THE THREE-PART BRAIN
Fish evolved brains composed of the cerebellum (which controls balance), the optic tectum (for sight) and the cerebrum (for awareness). The divisions persist in modern vertebrates

water. The optic tectum allows us to track objects with our eyes. The cerebrum is our center of self-awareness, memory and decision-making.

Neuroscientists can identify the main regions of the brain in every vertebrate, but just like small houses that start with a similar floor plan and are expanded in different ways, those brain regions have evolved into different shapes and sizes in different lineages. In some sharks, the cerebellum is larger than the other sections, while in salmon the optic tectum is larger. The vertebrates that moved on land—the tetrapods—tended to evolve larger cerebrums. In mammals, which first evolved 200 million years ago, the outer layer of the cerebrum expanded dramatically.

Biologists are investigating what evolutionary forces drove brains down these different paths. It appears that the brains of our ancestors changed in part because of a shift in their senses. Early mammals were dependent on their sense of smell, as reflected in the large bulge in skull fossils where the smell-interpreting part of the brain is located. Today many mammals still rely mainly on their sense of smell. Shrews dedicate 60% of their cerebral cortex to processing information from their noses. But our primate ancestors shifted toward sight. Primate eyes migrated from the sides to the front of the face, giving them powerful depth perception. And the primate brain began to change as well. A series of mutations allowed early primates to see a wider range of colors. They began to rely more on their eyes than their noses to find food. The brain regions that interpreted signals from their noses shrank, while the visual centers ex-

panded. This shift toward vision had a big impact on the social lives of our ancestors too. Primates evolved new centers in the brain that could quickly recognize other primates from the sight of their faces as well as figure out what they were feeling.

Reading faces is just one aspect of what scientists call the "social brain" of primates. Most species of primates live their entire lives in a group—sleeping together, searching for food together, escaping leopards and other predators together and sometimes even fighting off other groups of primates together.

Robin Dunbar, a psychologist at Oxford, has proposed that the increasing social complexity of primate life was a major force in the evolution of the species' brains. Compared to other mammals, primates have very big brains (and we humans have the biggest brains of all relative to our bodies). Dunbar hypothesized that natural selection favored big brains in animals that had complicated social lives.

To track the evolution of the primate brain, Dunbar began to measure what fraction of it was taken up by the cerebral cortex in each species. The bigger the average size of a social group in a species, the bigger that fraction of the brain. Human brain growth, Dunbar suggests, may have been boosted as our ancestors came together into ever bigger, ever more complex groups.

A larger brain and a more complex social life may have fostered the evolution of language, our ultimate social-networking widget. But our capacity for language did not emerge out of the blue. Our ability to speak depends on a set of brain regions. Those regions were already involved in language-like tasks in our an-

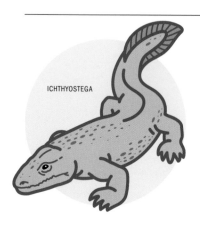

TETRAPODS
Creatures that move about on land needed a different brain from that of their watery forebears. Thus, they evolved larger cerebrums; in some species, these grew dramatically

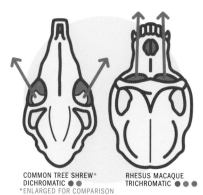

COMMON TREE SHREW*
DICHROMATIC ● ●
*ENLARGED FOR COMPARISON

RHESUS MACAQUE
TRICHROMATIC ● ● ●

A BETTER VIEW
Primates' eyes shifted to the front of the head, improving depth perception. We also became better at seeing colors. As we relied more on our sight, the scent regions of our brains shrank

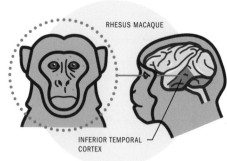

RHESUS MACAQUE

INFERIOR TEMPORAL CORTEX

WHO'S WHO
Primates' growing reliance on vision led to the growth of the inferior temporal cortex. This is the area that allows us to recognize other primates by face and intuit their feelings

cestors, as scientists have found by studying the brains of our primate relatives. Monkeys can make several different calls, and each has a distinct meaning (they may make one alarm call when snakes attack, for example, and another when the danger is a leopard).

Allen Braun and his colleagues at the National Institutes of Health recently investigated the parts of the brain that become active when monkeys hear these sounds. They had macaque monkeys listen to random noises as well as notes from musical instruments and the coos and screams of other macaques. Later, when the scientists compared the responses of the monkeys to the sounds, they discovered that the two sounds from macaques triggered regions of the brain that the others did not. Those regions turned out to be in the same location in the brain as language-processing regions. Braun and his colleagues proposed that before these regions processed human language, they processed simpler information that primates shared with one another.

Human language depends on more than just the existence of these regions; it also depends on their connections. An intricate bundle of nerve fibers, called the arcuate fasciculus, relays signals among the language-processing regions. When the arcuate fasciculus is damaged, people have a hard time reading words aloud and jumble the syllables in words as they speak.

James Rilling of Emory University and his colleagues recently conducted the first detailed comparison between the human arcuate fasciculus and the connections inside the brains of other primates. Before Rilling's research, scientists had dissected brains

Macaques process the calls of other macaques in a specialized region of the brain, separate from those that process other sounds. This is an early form of a language center, which grew vastly more complex in humans

to map these nerve fibers. Rilling was able to get a much more detailed picture with a technique called diffusion tensor imaging, which detects water molecules in nerve fibers. The work revealed that macaque monkeys, which branched off from our own ancestors 30 million years ago, have a simpler version of the arcuate fasciculus. Chimpanzees, which branched off only about 7 million years ago, have a much more intricate version. Humans just added on some extra connections to produce the full-blown arcuate fasciculus we have today.

Discoveries like Rilling's do not make our brain any less marvelous. It remains the most complex information-processing system in the world. But the growing body of research does, bit by bit, make the origin of the human brain a little less mysterious. ∎

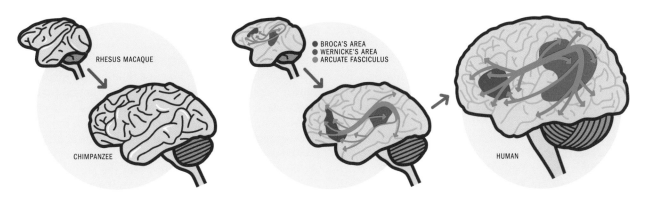

THE SOCIAL BRAIN
The larger the community group of a primate species, the larger that species' brain grew relative to body size. Humans' exuberant sociability may account for our particularly big brains

TALKING THE TALK
Macaques diverged from human ancestors 30 million years ago, and their brains have simple language regions. Chimps split off 7 million years ago and have better speech centers

TOP OF THE LINE
Nothing drives complex societies like language, and the key to human prolixity is the arcuate fasciculus, which weaves together the various brain regions that govern speech

Building a Brand-New Brain

It takes nine months to assemble the computer inside your head, and it takes a lot longer to program it properly. Genes play a big part, but so do experiences

BY J. MADELEINE NASH

RAT-A-TAT. RAT-A-TAT. IF SCIentists could eavesdrop on the brain of a human embryo 10 weeks after conception, they would hear an astonishing racket. Inside the womb, long before light first strikes the eye or the earliest images flicker through the cortex, nerve cells in the developing brain crackle with activity. Like teenagers with telephones, cells in one region are calling friends in another, and those cells are calling their friends, and they keep it up, says neurobiologist Carla Shatz of the University of California, Berkeley, "almost as if they were auto-dialing."

These staccato bursts of electricity arise from coordinated waves of neural activity that actually change the shape of the brain, carving mental circuits into patterns that over time will enable the newborn infant to perceive a father's voice, a mother's touch, a shiny mobile twirling over the crib. It took millions of years for human beings to acquire the brains we have today, but it takes only nine months for any one individual to grow any one brain. Even at birth, no brain is fully operational. Years of learning remain before all its wiring is complete.

A newborn's brain contains 100 billion neurons, roughly as many nerve cells as there are stars in the Milky Way. Also in place are a trillion glial cells, named after the Greek word for glue, which form a kind of honeycomb that protects and nourishes the neurons. But while the brain contains virtually all the neurons it will ever have, the hookups among them have yet to stabilize. Up to this point, says Shatz, "what the brain has done is lay out circuits that are its best guess about what's required for vision, for language, for whatever." Now it is up to neural activity—no longer spontaneous but driven by a flood of sensory experiences—to take this rough blueprint and progressively refine it.

The brain begins to take shape at about the third week of gestation, when a thin layer of cells in the embryo folds inward to give rise to a fluid-filled cylinder known as the neural tube. As cells in the neural tube proliferate at the astonishing rate of 250,000 a minute, the brain and spinal cord assemble in a series of tightly choreographed steps. Changes in the environment of the womb—whether caused by maternal malnutrition, drug abuse or a viral infection—can wreck the precision of the neural assembly line, sometimes leading to epilepsy, mental retardation, autism or schizophrenia.

What awes scientists is not that things occasionally go wrong but that so much of the time they go right. This is all the more remarkable, says Shatz, because the central nervous system of an embryo is not a miniature of the adult system but more like a tadpole that gives rise to a frog.

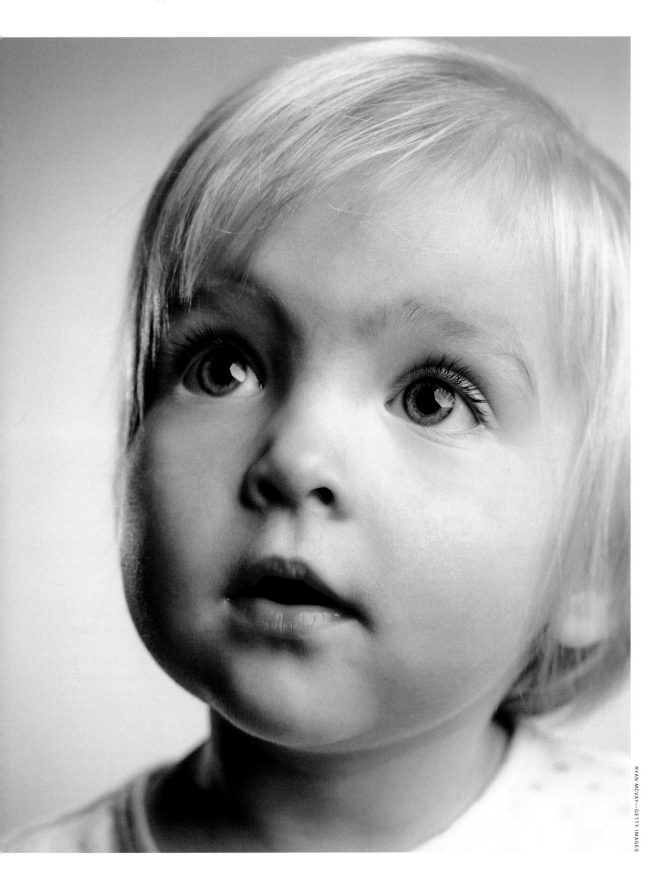

What biochemical magic underlies this metamorphosis? The instructions programmed into genes, of course. In the 1990s, for instance, scientists discovered a gene that helps steer the development of neurons in the spinal cord and brain. Like a strong scent carried by the wind, the protein encoded by the gene diffuses outward from the cells that produce it, becoming fainter and fainter. Columbia University neurobiologist Thomas Jessell has found that it takes middling concentrations of this potent morphing factor to produce a motor neuron and lower concentrations to make an interneuron, a cell that relays signals to other neurons.

Scientists have also identified genes that guide neurons in their long migrations. Consider the problem faced by neurons destined to become part of the cerebral cortex. Because they arise relatively late in the development of the mammalian brain, billions of them must push their way through dense colonies established by earlier migrants. "It's as if the entire population of the East Coast decided to move en masse to the West Coast," says Yale University neuroscientist Pasko Rakic.

But of all the problems the growing nervous system must solve, the most daunting is posed by the wiring. After birth, each of the brain's billions of neurons will forge links to thousands of others. First it must spin out a web of wirelike fibers known as axons (which transmit signals) and dendrites (which receive them).

What guides an axon is a "growth cone," a creepy, crawly sprout that looks like an amoeba. Scientists have known about growth cones since the early 20th century. What they didn't know until recently was that growth cones come equipped with the molecular equivalent of sonar and radar. Just as instruments in a submarine or an airplane scan the environment for signals, so molecules arrayed on the surface of growth cones search their surroundings for the presence of certain proteins.

Up to this point, genes have run the show. As soon as axons make their first connections, however, the nerves begin to fire, and what they do starts to matter more and more. The developing nervous system has strung the equivalent of telephone trunk lines between the right neighborhoods. Now it has to sort out which wires belong to which house, a problem that cannot be solved by genes alone but by what a baby experiences after birth.

Initially, a newborn can see, hear, smell and respond to touch, but only dimly. The brain stem, a primitive region that controls vital functions like heartbeat and breathing, is complete. Elsewhere the connections are wispy and weak. But over the first few months of life, the brain's higher centers explode with new synapses. By the age of 2, a child's brain contains twice as many synapses and consumes twice as much energy as an adult's.

Wiring the Brain for . . .

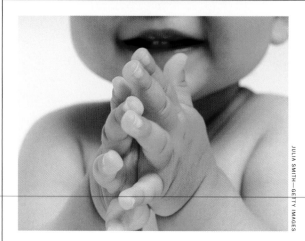

JULIA SMITH—GETTY IMAGES

FEELINGS

WHAT'S GOING ON: Among the first circuits the brain constructs are those that govern the emotions. At about 2 months of age, the distress and contentment experienced by newborns start to evolve into more complex feelings: joy and sadness, envy and empathy, pride and shame.

WHAT PARENTS CAN DO: Loving care provides a baby's brain with the right kind of emotional stimulation. Neglecting a baby can produce brain-wave patterns that dampen happy feelings. Abuse can produce heightened anxiety and abnormal stress responses.

WINDOW OF LEARNING: Emotions develop in increasingly complex layers. Teaching should grow more nuanced too.

This profusion of connections lends the growing brain exceptional resilience. Consider the case of Brandi Binder, a child who developed such severe epilepsy that surgeons had to remove the entire right side of her cortex when she was 6. Binder lost virtually all control over muscles on the left side of her body, the side controlled by the right side of the brain. Yet after years of therapy ranging from leg lifts to arithmetic and music drills, she became an A student, excelling at music, math and art—skills associated with the right half of the brain.

What wires a child's brain—or rewires it after physical trauma—is repeated experience. Each time a baby tries to touch a tantalizing object or gazes intently at a face or listens to a lullaby, tiny bursts of electricity shoot through the brain, knitting neurons into circuits. The results are those behavioral mileposts that delight and awe parents. Around the age of 2 months, the motor-control centers of the brain develop to the point that infants can suddenly reach out and grab a nearby object. Around the age of

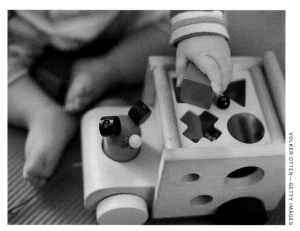

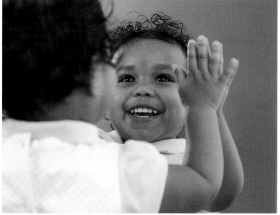

MOVEMENT

WHAT'S GOING ON: At birth, babies can move their limbs but in a jerky, uncontrolled fashion. Over the next four years, the brain progressively refines the circuits for reaching, grabbing, sitting, crawling, walking and running.

WHAT PARENTS CAN DO: Give babies as much freedom to explore as safety permits. Just reaching for an object helps the brain develop hand-eye coordination. As soon as children are ready for them, activities like drawing and playing a violin or piano encourage the development of fine-motor skills.

WINDOW OF LEARNING: Motor-skill development moves from gross to increasingly fine; step up the activities accordingly.

VISION

WHAT'S GOING ON: Babies can see at birth but not in fine-grained detail. They have not yet acquired the knack of focusing both eyes on a single object nor have they developed more sophisticated visual skills like depth perception. They also lack hand-eye coordination.

WHAT PARENTS CAN DO: There is no need to buy high-contrast black-and-white toys to stimulate vision. But regular eye exams, starting as early as 2 weeks of age, can detect problems that, if left uncorrected, can cause a weak or unused eye to lose its functional connections to the brain.

WINDOW OF LEARNING: Unless it is exercised early on, the visual system will not develop, so stimulation matters.

4 months, the cortex begins to refine the connections needed for depth perception and binocular vision. And around the age of 12 months, the speech centers of the brain are poised to produce language.

Critical players in this process are parents and other adults. Children who are physically abused early in life, for example, develop brains that are exquisitely tuned to danger. At the slightest threat, their hearts race, their stress hormones surge and their brains anxiously track nonverbal cues. Emotional deprivation early in life has a similar effect. University of Washington psychologist Geraldine Dawson monitored the brain-wave patterns of children born to mothers who had been given a diagnosis of depression. As infants, these children showed markedly reduced activity in the left frontal lobe, an area of the brain that serves as a center for joy.

Strikingly, not all the children born to depressed mothers develop aberrant brain-wave patterns. What accounts for the difference appears to be the emotional tone of the exchanges between mother and child. By scrutinizing hours of videotape, Dawson found that mothers who were disengaged, irritable or impatient had babies with sad brains. But depressed mothers who managed to rise above their melancholy, lavishing their babies with attention, had children with brain activity of a considerably more cheerful cast.

When is it too late to repair the damage wrought by physical and emotional abuse or neglect? For a time, at least, a child's brain is extremely forgiving. If a mother snaps out of her depression before her child is a year old, brain activity in the left frontal lobe quickly picks up.

Parents and teachers are rightly both humbled and thrilled by the power they have to shape the nature of the children for whom they care. The complexity of genes, neural tubes and axon growth may be far beyond most people's capacity to fully grasp. But the power of attention lovingly paid and lessons carefully taught is another matter entirely. ∎